"It is time for all those who love life to stand up and be heard. Dr. Bernard Jensen and Mark Anderson show us how to heal our planet and teach us how to find the path to personal and planetary health in their book *Empty Harvest*."

Bernie S. Siegel, MD
Author of *Love, Medicine & Miracles*

"In a day when it is cheap and easy to be a doomsday prophet, Empty Harvest shines like a bright beacon of hope and ecological sanity. While exposing the dire consequences of thinking we can grow healthy food with poisons, this excellent book defines positive alternatives, and demonstrates their power to restore us to true health. *Empty Harvest* lights the way toward living in harmony and happiness with the forces of life."

John Robbins
Author of *Diet for a New America*

"To think that human disease may simply reflect the quality of earth's topsoil is awe-inspiring...When a physician considers the causes of his patient's illness, it is too easy to blame a symptom. Reaching out for the quality of food consumed may be much closer to the cause of the disease. Anderson and Jensen lay out a picture of an Empty Harvest and propose constructive strategies to turn our emptiness around."

Jonathan Collins, MD
Editor-in-Chief, *Townsend Letter for Doctors*

"A formidable counterattack against the consipracy of commercial greed and its detriment to health...At long last, the true story of declining health in America has been told. *Empty Harvest* gets to the root of the problem...it should be required reading for the sincere physician and those seeking answers to their health problems."

Richard P. Murray, DC
Research Biochemist, Lecturer, and Nutritional Consultant

"An excellent book for physicians and lay persons alike. The section on special vitamin nutrient indications is especially useful and informative. The background material on mineralization is of special value and represents a new approach to an ever-increasing problem."

George Goodheart, DC
Developer of Modern Applied Kinesology

"Finally, a book is here that connects the whole cycle from soil to plants to animal/man and back to the soil again. In the landmark publication, *Empty Harvest* Dr. Bernard Jensen has joined with Mark Anderson, to produce an incredible indictment of the empty harvest of "modern" chemical agribusiness....*Empty Harvest* is not just another foreboding glimpse of the destruction around us. It is as refreshing as a spring rain and will germinate from the dormancy of hopelessness to a new and real hope for the future...This book is a form of nutrition..."

Review
The Organic Farmer

"*Empty Harvest* is not our first warning of ecological disaster, or the dangers from contamination of our food supply, but it is one of the most eloquent written in language anyone can understand, and with a message that is unmistakably clear. This is a book that deserves to be widely read."

Review
The Michigan Federation of Food Cooperatives Magazine

"This book is a wonderful potpourri of ecological words of wisdom for the body, soul, earth, atmosphere, planet and our minds...They have woven into the fabric of this wonderful reading material, the historical works of such nutrition greats as Dr. Weston Price, Dr. Royal Lee, and Dr. Harvey W. Wiley."

Catherine Frompovitch, PhD
Health Care Rights Advocates

"Jensen and Anderson have presented a factual and documented case for the concept of all disease being caused by malnutrition and immune-suppressing chemical toxicity, that every American should read.

Review
The Townsend Letter for Doctors

"The most significant book of the last quarter of the twentieth century. It is the core marrow of the knowledge of simultaneously healing the Earth and our bodies. My 35 years as a doctor has proven to me how true this book is. Every doctor, patient, farmer, food processor, grocery store and politician needs this information today."

D.A. Versendaal, DC
Developer of the Contact Reflex Analysis & Applied Trophology

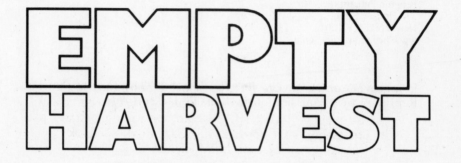

EMPTY HARVEST

UNDERSTANDING THE LINK BETWEEN OUR FOOD, OUR IMMUNITY, AND OUR PLANET

DR. BERNARD JENSEN
& MARK ANDERSON

AVERY
a member of Penguin Putnam Inc.

Paper sculpture on front cover by Blake Hampton.
Cover design by Rudy Shur and Martin Hochberg
In-house editor: Nancy Marks Papritz

Avery
a member of
Penguin Putnam Inc.
375 Hudson Street
New York, NY 10014
www.penguinputnam.com

Library of Congress Cataloging–in–Publication Data

Jensen, Bernard, 1908–
    Empty harvest : understanding the link between our food, our
immunity, and our planet / Bernard Jensen, Mark Anderson.
        p.   cm.
    Includes bibliographical references.
    ISBN 0–89529–558–X : $9.95
        1. Nutritionally induced diseases.   2. Health.   3. Nutrition.
4. Agriculture.   I. Anderson, Mark.   II. Title.
RA645.N87J46   1989
363.8—dc20   89–38643
                                                                          CIP

Printed in the United States of America

Contents

I dedicate this book to man's potential. What does it matter if we can walk on the Moon and visit Mars if we cannot control, or live in partnership with, the Earth of which we are a part and call our home.

—B.J.

Dedicated to
Dr. Royal Lee
Dr. Harvey Wiley
Major-General Sir Robert McCarrison
Dr. Weston Price
Sir Albert Howard
Dr. William Albrecht

They were unafraid of the bricks and mortar of scientific truth: the facts. They were all Three-Century Men. Born in the nineteenth century, they lived, worked, and achieved understanding in the twentieth century; but their foundational works will not be acknowledged or fully understood until the twenty-first century. Taken together, their applied wisdom could have created a twentieth century of planetary fulfillment, free of disease, in which all the kingdoms of the Earth lived in harmony.

Special dedication to my co-author, Dr. Bernard Jensen, who, in his eighty-first year, has been a tireless global teacher of the principles of wholeness and caring, and with whom it has been my honor to work.

—M.A.

Preface

The Earth is our Mother.

Though I now consider myself fortunate to know this truth, I must admit that learning it was to be the costliest lesson of my life.

When I was a young man, I thought that life was a bowl of cherries and the Earth was a cherry orchard. I believed I could keep filling my bowl and the Earth would continue to provide the cherries—without my ever having to give anything back.

It was only after near-fatal illness brought me to the brink of death that I began to understand the link between mankind and the planet Earth. This terrifying experience was to become the catalyst for my life's work in the healing arts; work which, today, spans more than fifty-five years and sixty-five countries.

I was twenty years old when doctors diagnosed my condition as bronchiectasis, a chronic inflammation of the lungs.

At that time, there was no cure. By living on foods that were nutritionally empty, overworking my mind and body daily at a dairy and, nightly, at chiropractic college, I made the foolhardy mistake of robbing Mother Nature. At the time of my illness, I had hit rock bottom; I had used up every gift that nature had given me and had given nothing in return.

It was only after consulting a Seventh Day Adventist physician that I realized there was a difference between a poor food regimen and a healthy one. This doctor declared that my disease was caused by nutritional deficiencies. He said I was "starving" myself with a diet of empty foods.

In its place, he prescribed a diet full of healthy foods. I combined this with breathing exercises given by Thomas Gaines, who once worked for the New York Police Department, and my condition improved. I began to gain weight, put several inches of flesh back on my chest, and found renewed energy. I was back on the road to health.

Because nutrition had helped save my life, I began to study foods. But I learned that one cannot really understand the value of foods without first studying the soil, what it is, and how it contributes to life and health. I learned about the value of specific foods from V. G. Rocine, a Norwegian homeopathic physician who had studied the findings of the European food chemists. I learned about the value of soil from William A. Albrecht, Ph.D., professor of agriculture at the University of Missouri.

Dr. Albrecht taught that unhealthy soil will yield unhealthy plants; and humans who subsist on plants grown in unhealthy soil will themselves grow weak. Albrecht taught that soil can be ruined by several processes—most of them involving man's interference—and that the crops grown on such land will not build healthy bodies. Though they may look like healthy crops and taste like healthy crops, they will be nutritionally deficient, Albrecht cautioned.

For this reason, consumers must not trust the appearance and taste of produce as a guide to its nutritional content. Modern farming may be capable of producing pretty crops. But nature alone can supply the nutrition within.

There are various ways in which soil becomes depleted of essential nutrients. Bad farming techniques can result in loss of topsoil through erosion. Growing the same crops on the same land year after year will rob the soil of nutrients. Misuse and overuse of chemical fertilizers and pesticides will kill not only bad, but good, forms of life in the soil, leaving only lifeless dust behind.

However, it is not necessary for soil to be wholly exhausted for it to impact our health in a negative way. For instance, if the soil is rich in most minerals but lacks calcium, food crops grown on it will lack calcium. Likewise, soil deficient in the micromineral boron will yield plants equally deficient in that micromineral, even if it is balanced in other ways.

Viewed individually, mineral deficiencies in these plants may not seem to be health threats. But, as we will learn in the pages that follow, the long-term deprivation of but a microscopic quantity of one essential nutrient in our diets alters the precise and vital balance of the body's chemicals. Ultimately, this results in symptoms that are the precursors to chronic or fatal disease.

Sadly, it appears that modern agriculture has outgrown its dependence on nature. While farmers in centuries past were forced to let dead fields lie fallow until the combined efforts of wildlife and rotting plants returned their fertility, modern farming technology allows us to ignore symptoms of soil exhaustion.

Incredible but true, today's high-tech farmers continue to douse dead land with antibiotic toxic chemicals that force green plants to grow against the will of a sickened Mother Earth. Her response in the face of this assault is fierce: An empty harvest.

During my years of study, I have learned that the soil is alive, that it needs to be fed properly just like any other living entity. It needs periodic rest if it is to continue to produce a rich harvest of nutritious food crops. Like all those we love and care for, Mother Earth deserves to be well fed and given the proper attention and rest. It is then that she will repay us by bringing forth fruit that is health-building.

In the years that followed my conversion from a sickly junk-food addict to healthy proponent of natural foods and organic farming, I became excited by the prospect of starting a sanitarium on a ranch where I could grow much of the food my patients would eat. By combining what I had learned from Rocine and Albrecht with Robert Rodale, publisher of

Organic Gardening magazine and owner of the Rodale Publishing empire, I was ready to give organic farming a try. The results? Great success.

At my Hidden Valley Ranch in Escondido, California, I took land, once used to grow alfalfa and graze cattle, and converted it, over a period of years, to a rich and productive organic farm.

The Ranch consisted of a flat valley flanked by boulder-strewn hills on two sides. I grew vegetables in the valley. Along one hillside were planted several varieties of grapes while on the other side was planted a fruit orchard. In the orchard we grew apricots, pears, plums, apples, peaches, nectarines, persimmons, figs, mulberries, kumquats, loquats, grapefruit, oranges, lemons, tangerines, and tangelos. In the rich, organic soil of the valley, we grew lettuce, carrots, beets, squash, corn, tomatoes, onions, radishes, melons, peas, beans, turnips, okra, artichokes, and more—often five to eight varieties of the same vegetable.

My fruit orchard became the dining room for birds from miles around. Eventually, I enclosed the whole orchard with chicken wire screen so we could have some of the fruit for ourselves. Although neighboring farms had as many fruit trees and berry bushes as we did, the birds left theirs alone and came to ours. Perhaps this was because we did not use any toxic insecticides, fertilizers, or manufactured chemicals. We had our own compost heaps and bought additional organic fertilizers as needed.

What the birds knew instinctively, the humans learned more slowly. One gentleman came to visit the Ranch often because he said it was the only place where he could get relief from persistent eye ulcers. Each time he returned home following a visit to the Ranch, the eye ulcers would return. I knew that this was because, once home, he would resume eating fruits and vegetables with chemical spray residues from his local supermarket instead of the clean, organically grown produce he ate while at the Ranch. When I persuaded the gentleman to plant his own organic garden at home, his eye ulcers never returned.

My experiences running the Ranch the organic way taught me that Mother Earth will reward us bountifully if we only treat her gently. Like our human reproductive systems, that of the Earth is delicate, and too much of a disturbance or imbalance can destroy her ability to bear fruit.

Happily, there are others who understand this truth. My co-author, Mark Anderson, is one of them. I met Mark at a recent Whole Health Institute Conference in Estes Park, Colorado, to which we were both invited. The workshop he gave there not only mirrored my own experience, but harmonized with it like a piano duet.

Mark told how the immune system of the human race is inextricably linked to the immune system of our planet. As long as the Earth, its topsoil, and its varied environments are healthy, Mark observed, the human race will be healthy. But when the Earth ails, the human race ails.

An interesting part of Mark's workshop at that conference was his reflection on the way native Americans had lived on this continent for several thousand years without disturbing its ecological balance or interfering with its ability to provide food, clothing, and other necessities for human survival. It was only after European settlers began to gorge themselves on the land's bounty without regard for replacing it, he reflected, that a downward spiral ensued.

Today, a little over two centuries since these settlers arrived on this continent, we have produced such toxic chemical pollution of our country's air, water, and soil, that there is real concern over our ability to clean it up.

In 1962, an unusual book, entitled *Silent Spring*, stirred a controversy in the United States and alerted many people that toxic chemicals threaten life on our planet. The book, written by Rachel L. Carson, is dedicated to the great physician and philosopher Albert Schweitzer, who said, "Man has lost the capacity to foresee and to forestall. He will end by destroying the earth."

The title, *Silent Spring*, is a word picture of a spring without bird songs. Birds eat plants sprayed with chemicals intended to kill insects. The birds die. The reader is left to question, *Who will be next?* The implications are clear.

With *Silent Spring*, Carson's contribution was not the presentation of a doomsday sermon. Rather it was the careful and scientific documentation of damage done by human hands to our planet's air, soil, rivers, and oceans, through the year 1960.

Now, nearly three decades later, we can make comparisons to judge whether progress has indeed been made. We have to realize that men and women were unable to destroy the world before the twentieth century because they did not have the technology with which to do it. But the twentieth century has been an era of chemicals, drugs, and nuclear radiation. Even without another world war, it is possible these days for the major world powers to destroy all life by poisoning the Earth—accidentally.

Mark Anderson and I have joined forces to write this book with the hope that it will guide our fellow inhabitants of this planet to a more harmonious and respectful relationship with our Mother Earth. To this end, my explanations of the relationship between soil and man lead the text in Part I. Mark's discussion about man, Earth, and immunity comprises Part II. In the Conclusion, I present various ways to help Mother Earth recover her health and fertility.

For years I have been a student of nature. I have tried to listen to what nature has said. I have tried to be sensitive to the needs of the soil, to the plant life, to the nature of nature. I have learned that when man departs from nature, opposes nature, or treats nature ignorantly or abusively, he does so at his own peril.

When we are able to accept the truth that this planet, the soil, the air, the water, and the entire universe are living systems, just as our bodies are composed of living systems, it becomes logical for us to live according to natural laws and processes that support and replenish those systems.

There is a fairy tale I often tell to relate the problem I perceive with modern agriculture. It goes like this:

There once were a couple of poor folks who discovered their goose laid eggs of gold. At first, they were delighted to take the eggs to town and get money to pay for the things they needed to buy. But, after a while, they became impatient and killed the goose so that they could get all the eggs inside at once. After doing so, they were shocked to find that there were no eggs inside the goose and, now that it was dead, there would be no more golden eggs.

Could we be exhibiting the same ignorance and greed with Mother Earth? By ignoring the creative life processes of which we are rightly a part and forcing her to produce against her will, we find our shortcuts leave us bankrupt. Like the foolish man and woman in the fairy tale, when we destroy nature to extract what we think we want in the short run, we are left with nothing in the end.

We must relearn how to "walk lightly on the land," as our native American ancestors taught. We must learn to love this planet and heed the message of the empty harvest. That is, in protecting the fate of the Earth Mother, we protect our fates as well.

Dr. Bernard Jensen
Escondido, California

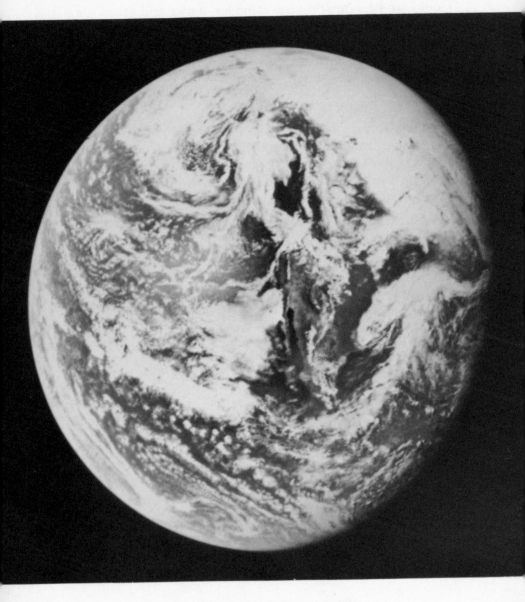

A View of Mother Earth From Space

As a net is made up by a series of ties, so everything in this
world is connected by a series of ties. If anyone thinks
that the mesh of a net is an independent, isolated thing,
he is mistaken.

Buddha

What befalls the earth befalls all the sons of the earth. . . .
This we know: the earth does not belong to man,
man belongs to the earth. All things are connected like
the blood that unites us all. Man did not weave the web
of life, he is merely a strand in it. Whatever he does to
the web, he does to himself.

Chief Seattle

We travel together, passengers on a little space ship,
dependent on vulnerable supplies of air and soil . . .
preserved from annihilation only by the care, the work,
and I will say the love, we give our fragile craft.

Adlai Stevenson

Part I

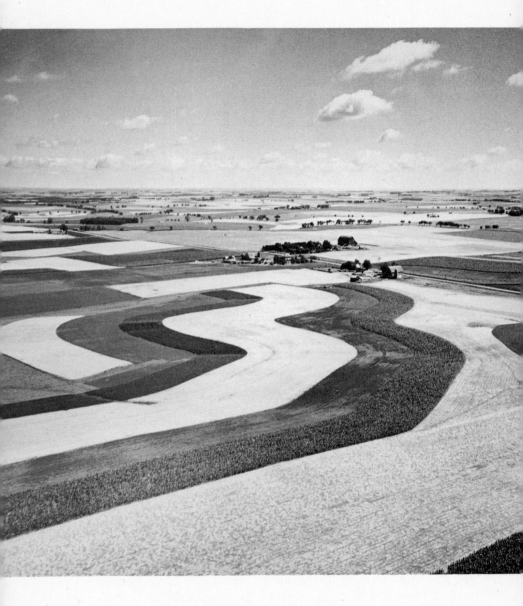

Lush Fields Belie an Empty Harvest

1
Soil and Civilization

Healthy soil is America's greatest natural resource. But few realize that the current state of widespread soil erosion in North America threatens our way of life. It may seem hard to believe, but only a few inches of topsoil stand between you, me, and starvation. Just what makes care of the topsoil so important? There are several things to consider.

First, soil is the medium for all plant life. What is popularly called topsoil is the rich, nutrient-laden cover of the Earth's crust from which food crops draw their sustenance. Underneath the topsoil there may be clay, shale, or rock—substances that do not support food crops. It is only in the precious shallow topsoil that plants are seeded, germinated, sprouted, nurtured, and grown. These plants serve as food for animals on the lowest ends of the food chain. Animals that eat these plants supply food to animals on the highest ends of the food chain.

Second, attention to topsoil is important because topsoil is easily exhausted from lack of care. The best farmers replenish the soil as it is farmed. Unfortunately, this practice has become an exception to the rule. Results of ignorance of proper agricultural methods can be seen in every country on Earth. Even in the Amazonian tropical rain forest, where many of us might assume that topsoil is extra rich due to the intense heat, humidity, and rapid decomposition of surrounding plants, topsoil exhaustion is epidemic. In this area of the world, farmers continue to practice a form of slash-and-burn agriculture. They cut down several acres of trees and vegetation, burn it, and then plant their crops. In a few seasons, the land is as barren and sterile as a desert. Then, they move on. Needless to say, this practice does not help the soil quality.

Third, care of topsoil is important because it is dependent on life around it to retain its own life-giving properties. One of the main reasons for the famine in East Africa today is lack of topsoil brought about by massive deforestation. At the turn of the century, 90 percent of Ethiopia's land was covered by forests. Less than a century later, not 5 percent of that forest remains. How did this occur? With the trees cut down for easy profit, the rain water—instead of soaking into the topsoil—rushed down the hillsides, flooded the valleys, and carried the earth off with it. The trees had shaded the soil, and the roots had acted as pumps, drawing water up near the surface of the ground, keeping the water table high. But now they were gone. Without tree roots to keep the water table high, the soil was exposed to sun, wind, and rain. It was baked dry, washed away into streams, rivers, and oceans, or simply blown away. Without soil in which to grow plants to feed animals and humans, mass starvation soon resulted.

Care of our forests cannot be overstressed. This is because the destruction of any kind of forest causes great imbalance in the planet's ecosystem. Trees are vitally important not only for soil stability but also because they give us our human breath, and we give them theirs. Trees release oxygen and consume carbon dioxide. Humans do the reverse.

Further, deforestation without replanting is a threat to nature because it kills non-hybrid progenitor trees and plants.

For instance, the progenitor of all coffee bean trees is from Ethiopia. If the last of these trees died from neglect, the hybrid species would become the ultimate source of coffee beans. But if the hybrid coffee bean trees around the world were then killed by some species-specific disease or agricultural malaise, there would be no original seed to fall back upon. Then, coffee bean trees—not to mention coffee breaks—would become extinct. While coffee is not a matter of life and death, this example of how biology impacts sociology is one that the Earth's inhabitants might do well to ponder.

THE LIMITS OF EROSION

Some soil erosion is natural. Wind picks up dust, and rain washes it away. Normally, nature can manage to replace the loss, slowly weathering sand and clay from rock, and mixing it with organic matter. But our destructive approach toward agriculture and development speeds erosion rates far beyond what nature can replace.

Highway construction, for instance, can accelerate erosion 200 times the natural rate. In just a matter of months, shopping-center development, surface mining, logging, and off-road vehicles can obliterate topsoil that nature took a thousand years to create—and needs a thousand years to replace.

Just how much damage has man done? In Iowa, topsoils that were once a foot deep today are less than six inches deep. Although it doesn't sound like much, six inches can be devastating. The United States Department of Agriculture estimates that a six-inch loss of topsoil, such as the current one in the southern Piedmont, is capable of reducing crop yields by 40 percent per year. Though crop loss and deforestation are bad enough, they are not the only soil erosion stories.

Soil erosion interferes with wildlife in many ways. When soil fertility is reduced, there is less life in the soil. That means less food for all animals—from the worms and insects to the birds that eat them to the larger animals that eat birds and, finally, to humans. Soil erosion kills water ecosystems, as well. The silt that accumulates in lakes because of runoff

causes the lakes to grow shallower. Then the weeds prolifer-
ate, choking off oxygen needed by fish. Fish die, and the
same negative sequence of events—only in an aquatic set-
ting—occurs.

My teaching and traveling experiences have made me
aware that people are not taught how intricately their lives
are woven with the life of their land. This ignorance is reflected in abusive agricultural methods. It is reflected in the
way people eat, accepting into their bodies foods grown on
sterilized, poisoned soils that have all too few nutrients to im-
part to the plant—or to them.

WE DON'T HAVE AS MUCH LAND AS WE THINK

Geologists say there are 58 million square miles of land surface on the Earth, but only 10 million square miles of this can
be farmed. It takes about two acres of land to feed one person
for a year. But, right now, there is only one acre per person,
and not all of this is good land. That is why, in my opinion,
about two-thirds of the people of the world go to bed hungry
every night.

Fortunately, the United States has enough land to feed its
people well. But there are still serious problems with the way
we use our land. More than half of the agricultural land of the
United States has been severely eroded or farmed incorrectly.
According to the United States Department of Agriculture, of
our current 421 million acres of productive farmlands, 97 million acres are eroding at more than twice the "tolerance"
level—the level at which soil can be replaced naturally. Another 89 million acres are eroding at one to two times that
tolerance level. In all, nearly 40 percent of our farmlands are
losing topsoil.

Ecologist Gene Logsdon wrote, "The fall of almost every
civilization is largely on account of raping natural resources
until all the easy profit goes out of them." By the 1930s, most
of the "cream" had been skimmed off of American soils, and
diminished crops of mineral-deficient vegetables, fruits, and
grains began to appear. Interestingly, chronic, degenerative
diseases began to escalate at this time, as well—arthritis, diabetes, cancer, lupus, osteoporosis, and dental caries.

TISSUE-INTEGRITY AND WELLNESS

Over a sixty-year period, I have witnessed the deterioration of our planet and its life-giving systems, and the degenerative effect this has had on people.

My observations have led me to conclude that we should understand that people with nutritional deficiencies and toxic accumulations are not just "less healthy" than other people. We cannot separate the body from the mind or from the spirit. Any person with impaired wellness at the physical level is, to some degree, impaired mentally and morally. The mind does not work as well. The strength of will that is so important in living a life of integrity is lowered.

In fact I have never failed to notice, though I loved all my patients, that the sickest among them were the most mentally ill, morally weak, and emotionally imbalanced.

Also aware of this relationship was my late friend, J. I. Rodale, of the Rodale natural foods publishing empire. He often said he believed there was a correlation in the fact that my ancestral home of Denmark boasted two dubious world records: Number One in both its use of artificial fertilizers and its annual suicide rate. Rodale said he felt there was a connection between Denmark's dead soil and its dead people.

But, luckily, the effects of dead soil can be reversed. As I taught my patients to cleanse and correctly feed themselves, as they restored themselves to physical health, my greatest joy was in witnessing the mental, moral, and emotional recovery that also occurred in them.

WE ARE MADE OF THE DUST OF THE EARTH

The Bible says that man is made of the dust of the Earth. The same chemical elements found in soil make up our bodies. The only difference between the two is that the human molecular structure is more complex. Human bodies require nutrition found in the form of plants, meat, milk, and eggs.

But all animals get their food directly or indirectly from plants, and all plants get their food from the soil. Therefore, mineral-deficient soil may be one of the greatest original sources of disease in the world today. According to D. W. Cavanaugh, M.D., of Cornell University, "There is only one major disease and that is malnutrition. All ailments and afflictions to which we may fall heir are directly traceable to this major disease." Simply stated, food crops grown on depleted soil produce malnourished bodies, and disease preys on malnourished bodies.

A few of the trace minerals necessary for plant health and resistance are: magnesium, zinc, iron, copper, calcium, boron, manganese, molybdenum, cobalt, and chromium. But the absence of one element from the soil can cause great health problems. For instance, if inorganic cobalt is missing in the soil, the plant cannot absorb it and convert it to organic cobalt. Without organic cobalt, the human body cannot manufacture vitamin B_{12}. When we don't get enough vitamin B_{12}, we can't assimilate iron properly or make strong red blood cells; we become anemic. Anemic people become weak, depressed, and vulnerable to disease.

THE ELEMENTS OF MANKIND

I want you to have a look at Table 1.1, the German chemist Wilhelm Koenigs' famous list of chemicals that compose the human body. I want you to consider briefly what happens to your body when you are missing one or more of these elements.

Table 1.1   Koenigs' Analysis of Chemical Elements in an Average Mature Male

Element	Percent	Element	Percent
Oxygen	59.0	Potassium	.1
Carbon	23.0	Sodium	.1
Hydrogen	9.0	Fluorine	.1
Calcium	2.0	Magnesium	.1
Nitrogen	2.5	Silicon	.1
Phosphorus	2.3	Iron	.1
Chlorine	1.0	Iodine	.003
Sulfur	.2	Manganese	trace

When the body lacks one or more chemical element, the tissue structure is weakened, the cell function is impaired, and health problems can develop. The reason for this is nutrients combine in the body to form such critical materials as hormones, enzymes, and proteins. If the body is missing zinc and chromium, for instance, the pancreas cannot properly manufacture the hormone insulin. The inability of the pancreas to manufacture insulin results in diabetes, a degenerative condition in which the tissues are unable to obtain sugar from the blood.

A shortage of one mineral may cause more damage in one organ than another because of differences in chemical composition of some of our organs and tissue structures. A potassium shortage, for example, will affect every tissue in the body a little, but it will harm the heart muscle more than any other tissue. This is because potassium acts as a heartbeat regulator. A deficiency of potassium can result in racing of the heartbeat, called *tachycardia*.

Let's look at some of the other organs and tissues, and consider their nutrient needs. Table 1.2 shows some specific components of specific body organs and tissues.

Suppose the liver was deprived of zinc, selenium, sulfur, and iron. The liver would then be sluggish, slow in its function, defective in its performance, or weak in its ability to defend itself or to repair damaged tissue. The liver's job is to manufacture thousands of enzymes, manufacture bile for the digestion of fats and oils, process many nutrients into usable forms, detoxify the blood and bowel, and store sugar for energy. Having this immense agenda 24 hours a day, 365 days a year, for potentially more than 100 years, its need for the nutrients out of which it manufactures what it needs to accomplish all its tasks cannot be overstated. The minerals, amino acids, and vitamins the liver needs are supposed to come from plants which, in turn, should get them from the soil.

So we see how our bodies can become vulnerable in a particular organ or system if the diet is deficient in the natural chemical elements needed to nourish those particular tissues. That is why a disease may settle into one part of the body rather than another. Or, if you notice that some of the same

Table 1.2 Some Chemical Components
of Specific Body Organs and Tissues

Organ or Tissue	Components
Blood	calcium, cobalt, copper, iron, potassium, sodium, zinc
Blood Vessels	copper, magnesium, rutin, silicon
Bones	calcium, copper, fluorine, magnesium, manganese, phosphorous, silicon
Bowel	calcium, chlorine, fluorine, iodine, iron, potassium, sodium
Brain, Nerves	calcium, iodine, manganese, magnesium, phosphorous, potassium, silicon, sodium, sulfur
Heart	calcium, iron, magnesium, phosphorous, potassium
Joints	iron, manganese, sodium
Kidneys	calcium, chlorine, fluorine, iron, magnesium, potassium, silicon, sodium
Liver	iron, magnesium, potassium, selenium, sulfur, zinc
Lungs	calcium, manganese, phosphorous
Skin, Hair, Nails	calcium, copper, fatty acids, manganese, silicon, sodium, sulfur, zinc
Spleen	copper, fluorine, iron, magnesium, manganese, potassium, sodium

chemical elements feed several organs, you will understand that all of them can be affected by the same deficiencies.

Usually, the chemical deficiency (and later symptoms of disease) affects inherently weak tissue, not strong normal tissue. Strong tissue more effectively assimilates the chemical elements it needs than does inherently weak tissue. The inherently weak tissue is not able to absorb nutrients nor dispose of waste as effectively as does strong tissue.

WHAT STANDS IN OUR WAY

We cannot appreciate enough the importance of our relationship with the land, with soil. This is particularly so today, the era of artificial chemicals, artificial foods, and the abundance of artificial materials on which we have come to depend in place of real dirt and the living food crops it produces.

Our dependence on artificial, man-made products interferes with our relationship with the soil and the natural world in general. More and more of us are growing up with this dependency on artificial materials, making it increasingly difficult to maintain an awareness of our true "roots," and the true origins of health.

In addition to this, the availability of drugs, chemicals, and radiation gives us the power to self-destruct, individually as well as collectively. For the sake of those who may not yet be aware, and for the sake of young people whose education lacks such knowledge, the following is an explanation of just exactly why these artificial materials interfere with our health and well-being, and threaten the future of our children and this planet.

ARTIFICIAL CHEMICAL FERTILIZERS

These are fertilizers manufactured from petroleum-based chemicals, devoid of trace minerals. Artificial iron and magnesium are added because they are known to be essential, but other needed trace elements are generally neglected.

The problem with artificial chemical fertilizers is that they cannot be integrated into soil or plant life in the same way that bio-organic chemicals can. In a natural environment, life is renewed as dead vegetation decomposes and feeds the microbial life in the soil. Animals die, and their carcasses are broken down by predators, bacteria, insects, and so forth until they, too, become part of the soil. In contrast, most artificial chemical fertilizers are acid salts that burn their way through the soil, destroy its balance, and create imbalance by killing microbial life.

Most pesticides cause cancer by changing the genetic structure of humans and animals. They have been used for so long and in such heavy concentrations that our ground water is now contaminated with them. The United States Environmental Protection Agency (EPA) found that by the 1970s the water supplies of many cities and towns were contaminated and unsafe because of polluted ground water. For example, recent tests of the drinking water of the city of New Orleans, Louisiana produced no fewer than sixty-six foreign chemicals.

These chemicals kill most of the microorganisms and worms in the topsoil, causing an even more unhealthy soil condition. They trickle down through the ground into the underground water supply. Meanwhile, insects are developing immunity to insecticides so that more and more powerful sprays have to be introduced. It is a frightening but undeniable fact to ponder that most modern-day farms have at least one shed or storage room with enough poison in it to wipe out everyone in a city the size of Los Angeles.

Many agricultural chemicals have been proven to cause cancer, genetic damage, and nerve and brain damage. One of the alarming signs supporting this fact is the increase in birth defects since World War II. This is especially obvious in migrant workers and farm hands who work in the fields and directly expose themselves to these chemicals.

DDT: MAN-INVENTED MOLECULE

From 1947 to 1960, pesticide production increased from 259,000 thousand pounds per year to nearly 6.4 million pounds. In 1948, Paul Miller of Switzerland won a Nobel Prize for his discovery of chlorophenothane, dichlorodiphenyltrichloroethane, commonly known as *DDT,* one of the most deadly carcinogenic insecticides known to man. It was banned from the United States in the late 1960s because of massive public outcry following record-breaking sales of the book *Silent Spring* by Rachel Carson. DDT had already caused great damage to the environment, being found in the livers of ocean fish thousands of miles from where it could possibly have been used. It is found in the tissue of penguins in the North Pole. It has found its way into dairy products, fruits, and vegetables throughout the United States, and has contaminated the entire food chain. Although the United States no longer uses it, we manufacture it and sell it abroad where it is not yet banned. Then we get it back on foods imported from Third World countries such as Mexico.

DDT is a class of deadly insecticide known as a "chemical of organic synthesis." Like the insecticides heptachlor, chlordane, and 2, 4-D, DDT has no counterpart in nature. It is a completely *man-invented molecule*, so normal environmental process does not break it down. It can reside in full toxicity for thousands of years in the water and soil.

EFFECTS ON AQUATIC ECOSYSTEMS

From north to south, on the Pacific and Atlantic coasts, the deadly poisons spilling off our lands into the oceans are infecting the harvest of the sea. It is no wonder that news reports frequently focus on beached whales and dolphins. They lay helplessly trapped on the shore as if trying to escape from the toxic soup that was once their pristine wilderness.

Aquatic pollution is evident in other ways, as well. Fish caught by commercial fishing boats off the Los Angeles area coast have four times higher toxin levels than fish from the San Diego offshore area. Toxic concentrations of chlordane, mercury, and toxaphene, are found in the flesh of fish from the Sacramento River Delta. Why? Because the runoff from the large agricultural regions of California affects mainly those areas where the runoff washes into the oceans.

Shellfish from the state of Maine are relatively clean because chemical agriculture is only a small business in this region. But in Maryland's busy ports along the Chesapeake Bay, shellfish are highly toxic. Sadly, Maine's shellfish are the exception. From Puget Sound in Washington State to Boston Harbor in Massachusetts, fish are often too contaminated to risk eating these days.

There are alternatives for fish-eaters. Commercially grown fish are generally safe, as are fish taken from cold mountain streams. But in our inland waterways, such as the Great Lakes, the EPA has alerted sports fishers that the fish they catch will be diseased with liver tumors and other sure signs of toxic contamination, results of waste dumping and acid rain in the industrial heartland of America.

RECOMMENDATIONS AND REFLECTIONS

The best way to ensure that your food is "clean" is to purchase produce, grains, poultry, fish, and meat from natural
food stores that sell toxin-free products. But don't take anything for granted. Ask questions of their produce buyers.
Find out how they know the produce is free of pesticides.
Ask to see proof.

As one who has found nature to be a reliable guide toward
health and wholeness, I believe that our farming methods
have taken us further from nature, drawing us deeper and
deeper into a toxic way of life. We are producing less nutritious food at the highest cost in history while United States
farmers are going bankrupt. We are saturating our bodies
with drugs to try to stop disease and saturating the Earth
with chemicals to try to stop insects and plant diseases.
Something must change if we do not want to go in the direction of disease and death.

We have to understand that whether toxic material is buried on land, dumped directly into rivers, or put into the atmosphere, it ends up in our soil, ground water, and oceans.
The Earth is no different from the human body in that it is a
closed system. If you poison one area, it soon travels to another area. A Kansas farmer can apply a poisonous chemical
to his plants and, over the course of time, that poison may
find its way into the schoolhouse lunch of a child in Pennsylvania, or into the liver of a penguin in the North Pole.

NUCLEAR RADIATION

The consequences of a nuclear accident or toxic outbreak can
affect several generations and disrupt the lives of people
thousands of miles from the source of contamination. For ten
days, radioactivity spewed into the atmosphere from the
Chernobyl Nuclear Power Plant in the Ukranian portion of
the Soviet Union. On Saturday, April 26, 1986, Soviet planes
dropped lead, sand, and boron onto the fire created by a
meltdown in the reactor core. Meanwhile, 50,000 people were
evacuated from the area. Two days later, levels of radioactivity
in Sweden were measured as high as 100 times normal. The

long list of these harmful substances included isotopes of krypton, xenon, iodine, cesium, and cobalt. The first Soviet news release about casualties came the next day, acknowledging 2 people dead and 197 hospitalized. Western scientists estimated that every unprotected human being within eighteen miles of the explosion would die within a few hours, while those as far as sixty miles downwind from the accident would die eventually as a direct result of radiation exposure. No one would be able to enter the immediate area for three to five years.

The governments of France, Finland, and Great Britain ordered evacuation of their citizens from the Kiev area. When they had returned to their countries, tests on these people revealed small amounts of radioactivity in their thyroid glands. None was found in their lungs or digestive systems. This is because the body treats the mutant radioactive iodine like the nutrient iodine. The thyroid uses nutrient iodine to make the hormone thyroxin, which prevents goiter. Polish children were given iodine solutions to drink, so their thyroids would not assimilate the radioactive iodine from Chernobyl. People in Tokyo, Japan were advised not to drink rainwater until further notice.

Experts predicted that the radioactive iodine would be nearly gone a month after the accident, but that the radioactive cesium and strontium would be dangerous for hundreds of years. Medical advisors have warned that for the next thirty years, the incidence of cancer in all the areas of Russia and other countries that received dangerous levels of exposure to radioactivity would skyrocket. This has begun to occur even faster than the rate first predicted.

Common sense tells us that we would not be facing such death-dealing accidents if we were not playing with such deadly substances as radioactive materials. Most people are aware that these are dangerous substances, but most may not understand why.

WHAT RADIATION IS AND WHAT IT DOES

Radioactive substances such as cobalt-60, iodine-131, and cesium-137 emit radiation in a manner something like X-rays, which pass through the body unnoticed and unfelt. However, this radiation is of such energy that it is able to knock off electrons from the chemical elements that make up our body cells. This process is called free-radical degeneration, and my co-author, Mark Anderson, considers it further in the next section. The removal of electrons damages the protein of the body and the genes. The worst damage is to cells that reproduce most rapidly—the cells of the ovaries, testes, bone marrow, bowel, and skin.

The standard unit of measurement for radiation is the *rem*, standing for "roentgen equivalent in man." This is the dose of radiation it takes to produce the same amount of biological damage as one roentgen of X-ray or gamma radiation. The dose of radiation to which a person is exposed has differing effects. For example, a blast of 5,000 rem kills right away. While not fatal at first, anything over 1,000 rem will cause death sooner or later.

Rem are measured per hour (similar to miles per hour) so that exposure to 200 rem for five hours would add up to 1,000 rem, a lethal level that causes death within days. The normal background level for radiation on the Earth's surface varies from place to place and depends on climate, altitude, and latitude; but the range is generally from as low as 10 millirem (thousandths of a rem) to more than 200 millirem. This is due to natural radiation from the Earth and from fallout accumulated on the Earth's surface since the first atomic bomb tests in the 1940s, including nuclear power plant accidents that have occasionally released radioactivity.

Radioactivity is, by and large, a long-term and very dangerous pollutant. It settles in water, soil, and plant life. It is found in the flesh of birds, wildlife, and domestic animals, and it travels up the food chain through air, water, animals (meat and milk), fish, vegetables, and fruit. It is both carcinogenic and mutagenic, able to cause genetic damage that results in deformed or otherwise abnormal offspring.

Radiation damage to individuals varies so widely that one person can die from a dose that leaves another person unharmed. From the same dose of radiation, one person may develop cancer in two years while another develops cancer in seventeen years. Different kinds of radioactive chemicals may concentrate in different parts of the body after ingestion.

SPECIFIC EFFECTS OF RADIOACTIVE ELEMENTS

Iodine-131 gathers in the thyroid gland, where its radiation can trigger genetic damage that gives rise to cancer decades after exposure, even though it has a half-life of eight days and is mostly gone from the body in two months. (The half-life of a radioactive chemical is the time it takes for the amount of radioactivity to drop to half its original level. Radioactive elements, like clocks, tend to "wind down" over a period of time.)

The whole body is affected by krypton-85, with a half-life of nearly eleven years. Cancers such as leukemia may appear in as little as two years after exposure to krypton-85. Cesium-137 also affects the whole body, but especially the liver and spleen. Its half-life is thirty years. Barium-140, with a half-life of 12.8 days, collects in the bones. Tumors may develop in from twenty to thirty years.

Radiation sickness develops in those exposed to radiation levels of, for example, 150 rem in one week's time. That would be the accumulated radiation from a little less than one rem per hour. Radiation sickness starts with loss of appetite, nausea, and diarrhea the first week, and may disappear the second week. Then, high fever, weight loss, and fatigue develop. Damage to the radiation-sensitive cells of the small intestine block assimilation of nutrients, and the white blood cell count drops quickly (immune system degeneration).

British physician Alice Stewart has spent much of her life investigating the connection between low-level radiation and higher cancer risks. Most doctors have stopped using fetal X-rays since Stewart's work showed that a significant increase in leukemia was found in the children of mothers who had prenatal X-rays taken. She has said she believes that the effects of background radiation coupled with exposure to X-rays may cause most childhood cancers.

RISKS OF FOOD IRRADIATION

What about food irradiation as an alternative to chemical preservatives? Let's take a look. Food irradiation is done with gamma rays from cobalt, which are capable of causing genetic change and mutation just like radioactive elements. Some scientists say that irradiation can cause chemical changes in food that could destroy nutrients and create carcinogens.

The Food and Drug Administration (FDA) tried to get irradiated foods approved and sold throughout the United States in 1989. However, due to overwhelming public rejection, grocery chains, afraid of alienating their customers, are refusing to sell irradiated produce. (Imported foods may still be irradiated, such as spices and herbs.) This public support has, for now, succeeded in blocking the use of irradiation as a food preservative technique in America. Our vigilance will keep it that way.

RADON GAS

In recent years, the EPA investigated and found the health danger posed by *radon gas* to be very real in the United States. The deadly nature of radon was first discovered several decades ago when uranium miners began to develop lung cancer. In a recent article in *American Health* magazine, "Living Room Lung Cancer," radon was implicated in 5,000 to 20,000 lung cancer deaths a year. Dr. Jacob Fabricant, chairman of the National Academy of Sciences Research Council committee on the biological effects of ionizing radiation, recently reported the conclusion of a three-year study of radon: Exposure to high levels of radon increases the risk of lung cancer, especially in smokers.

What is radon? Radon is a radioactive gas formed by the natural breakdown of the element radium. It is colorless, odorless, and tasteless, seeping up through the ground until it enters the air, or enters buildings through sewage pipes or foundation cracks. Outdoors it is harmless because it is so quickly diluted and dispersed. By contrast, inside a building, it can concentrate to deadly levels.

The danger of developing cancer from radon is greatest in well-insulated, tightly "weatherproofed" homes during winter months, especially in areas of the country where radon gas levels are naturally high. These areas include the expanse between Reading, Pennsylvania and northern New Jersey, and the Colorado plateau in the Rocky Mountains. Based on its studies, the EPA claims that more than 7.5 million

American homes may now contain dangerous levels of radon gas.

You can buy home radon tests in hardware stores or by mail for as little as ten or fifteen dollars. *Buyers Up,* a consumer group affiliated with Ralph Nader, offers a two-dollar guide to many radon test kits and labs rated for quality and convenience. (Write P.O. Box 33487, Washington, DC 20033–0487.)

Corrective steps include sealing cracks in basement floors and installing home ventilation systems. Costs range from three hundred to one thousand dollars.

A SILENT SPRING IS JUST AROUND THE CORNER

So, what is new since *Silent Spring* was published in 1962? There are half a million chemicals now in use. Ten thousand new chemical products are marketed each year. Pesticide use in the United States has more than doubled.

We have continued to pollute the atmosphere. As a result the "holes" in the earth's atmospheric ozone layer have grown wider. We have ignored non-polluting automotive technology that would eliminate automobile pollution.

The endangered species list has continued to grow, forests are burning, weather patterns are changing. This is causing more droughts and tornados. On and on the list goes. The statistics are all available. The broadcast and print media present these facts to us daily. Naturalists, environmentalists, and animal protection groups fight hard every day to gain a few victories over the onslaught of destruction.

THEN AND NOW

How far have we come since 1962? We would like to be optimistic and cite the victories and accomplishments. Certainly there have been some. But in order for us to bring the balance and health needed for the survival of this planet and humankind, we will have to go much further and take urgent steps. We no longer have the leisure time with which to carry out a ten- or twenty-year plan of restoration. Each of us must become dedicated to protecting what natural balance and health is left in us and in our planet. Each of us must play a part to increase balance and health in whatever way is possible. Those who begin by feeding their own bodies with good food usually find that their newfound health gives them the energy to help others. We begin to make ourselves heard in small ways, from placing demands on the grocer for safe, nutritious food, to speaking out for natural values and the future of our planet. We learn how to heal ourselves of disease and are then able to educate our children.

A clean environment is the foundation of life on this planet. It is the basis for health in every organ, gland, and tissue in the body. Every cell in our bodies depends, directly or indirectly, for life and health on its relationship with the external environment.

Until the past century, planet Earth was relatively pure and free of toxic chemicals. Beginning with the Industrial Revolution and during this Technological Age, man has violated virtually every law of nature. In doing so, he has weakened the Earth, the source of all his livelihood. As a result, man's health on all levels—physical, moral, mental, social—is now weak and compromised. This compromise manifests itself in escalating disease, confusion, and violence.

While the situation is dire, should fear be the correct catalyst for change? I don't think so. For fear is a disease in itself—a disease of the mind. Therefore, it is not out of fear, but courage, that mankind will be most effective in restoring health and harmony to this planet. Nature's call is clear. Now, we need only to join forces and act.

Part II

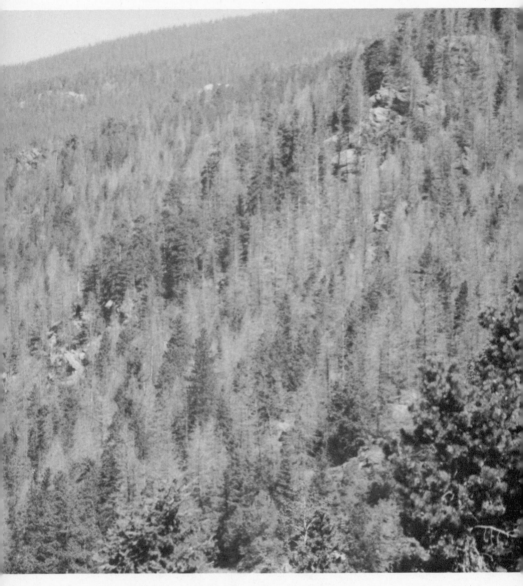

Watching Our Forests Die Without Understanding the Consequences

2

Man, Earth, and Immunity

I brought a sample of what may be some of the most ideal soil on the planet Earth to a lecture I gave recently. The soil came from my minerally enriched organic garden in Fort Collins, Colorado. After a great deal of work, it is among the most balanced, trace-mineral-rich soil you can find anywhere. I asked the doctors attending the lecture to touch the soil and hold it in their hands to experience direct contact with a high-quality soil, a soil exquisitely rich in minerals, biological precious metals.

When they touched the soil, that "touch" symbolized the first lesson we need to learn in strengthening our immune system: Our individual immune systems are inescapably linked to the planet Earth, of whose substance we are made. The entire planet Earth, the complete geosphere, has its own functioning immune system, a self-protecting, regenerating, healing system. When we are not integrated in that system, or we harm that system, the inevitable result is our own degeneration.

As the soil passed from hand to hand, we acknowledged that this is the most valuable commodity on Earth from which comes all the blessings that life bestows on mankind. There is no blessing that anyone has ever received that was not linked to the Earth, even if it came from the Sears catalog.

What we will explore together in this book is the interwoven fabric of the living immune system that encompasses all life within, on, and above the surface of the planet Earth. Viewed as such, a picture of wholeness emerges and we, as life's crowning creation, will see our remarkable role in rebuilding and preserving the global immune system.

THE IMMUNE SYSTEM: AN INTERNAL ALLIANCE

The subject of the human immune system, partly because of the worldwide epidemic of Acquired Immune Deficiency Syndrome (AIDS), is receiving wide coverage in the press these days, stirring a popular movement of concern and interest. However, the importance of the immune system should be nothing new for any serious health professional. In the early days of learning about physiology and biochemistry, one realizes that the immune system is not so much a system in the usual sense of body systems, like the skeletal system, the respiratory system, the reproductive system, where you can analyze and quantify and qualify the specific organs involved.

For example, in the respiratory system, we talk primarily about the lungs or the bronchial passageways. However, what we have with the immune system, to the dismay of specialists who love to divide the body into tiny specialized sections, is an alliance and a relationship, an integrated coalition of organs that works intersystem-wise to protect the body and to inform the body what belongs to it and what does not.

Like immigration or customs officials, the immune system determines what is allowed in the body (the country) and what must be deported. It has a remarkably sophisticated means of discerning this. This internal immune alliance includes the thymus gland (part of the endocrine system), the lymph nodes (lymphatic system), the spleen, the bones, the nervous system, the hypothalamus, and the brain. The major commonalty of this alliance we call "the immune system" is this: that all the allies manufacture their immune substances out of nutrients. These nutrients are vitamins, amino acids, minerals, trace elements, and essential fatty acids.

When we look at the global ecological travesty that we are in, we see too that the immune system of mankind is ominously jeopardized. We tend to think of the jeopardy in terms of some very special areas, the popularized media "items" such as AIDS. After all, the World Health Organization (WHO) forecasts that 75 million people are going to die from this immune system disease. But doesn't all life-threatening disease involve a collapse of the immune system? The National Cancer Institute predicts that one of every three Americans will be afflicted with a form of cancer in their lifetime. Thirty percent is the exact figure. One out of three. A collapse of the immune system. Though rare in the last century, cancer and heart disease are today's leading causes of death. Chronic degenerative diseases such as diabetes, arthritis, and lupus, which also reveal the collapse of the immune system, appear to be virtually out of control.

Yet, during the earlier part of this century, medical science gave us the highest hopes with the new "wonder drugs," antibiotics. It seemed that we finally had infectious disease under control. However, this was a false hope, a false god, who, during this last part of the century, has failed us, while driving more rational, natural approaches into the scientific underground.

In order to discuss the human immune system, let's look at the larger immune system of planet Earth. For, the two are like Siamese twins, connected at birth.

FROM UNNATURAL TO ANTI-NATURAL

As a culture, we are not just unnatural—it is deeper. We are anti-natural. One of the reasons that I sense such a kindred spirit with the native North American people is not only the romantic image I have of a beautiful people and how they lived, but more so because of a very scientific evaluation: Here was a people who inhabited this continent for thousands of years before the white man came, a people who had very actively lived on this land, used it for everything they needed and wanted, *and when the European settlers began arriving in the sixteenth century it was still in pristine condition after thousands of years of their use.* In the modern vernacular, this land was in "showroom condition" after thousands of years of use. (Would you rather buy a piece of land from an American Indian or from a modern farmer?)

The water was absolutely pure. You could stop anywhere and drink it, as long as it was flowing. The land, no matter where you went, was fertile. If a seed fell out of your pocket, a plant would grow. The trees and the forests were everywhere. An Iroquois chief told me that in his lore and legends of the Iroquois Nation they speak of how a squirrel could run from the Atlantic Ocean to the Father of the Great Waters, the Mississippi, and never touch the ground, leaping tree branch to tree branch. The Iroquois gave directions by noting "grandfather trees" as landmarks.

Here was a people so in tune with the Earth, its immune system and their own were so integrated, that, when the white man arrived here, he found an unspoiled, perfectly integrated, whole ecosystem where mineral, microbial, vegetable, insect, atmospheric, animal, and human kingdoms coexisted in balance. But, in a matter of a few hundred years, through wholesale exploitation and plain stupidity, the land lay decimated.

Clear cutting of forests and depletion of the soil began immediately by settlers. To date, about 260 million acres of American forests have been cleared for meat production. The vast majority of grain we grow is for livestock feed. A poisoning campaign, begun in the 1800s, and progressive depletion and demineralization of the soil have put North America within seven or eight inches of barren desert. Americans are not the only offenders, however. Figure 2.1 illustrates the effects of man's neglect on the Earth as a whole.

What we have done to the soil and the disregard we have shown for it is a travesty. We have watched it become wasted, poisoned, sterilized, and eroded, thus weakening our own immune system to the most dangerous level, which is why we need to begin right away to reverse the damage caused during the last century.

Although the popular ecology movement grabs an occasional headline, what our political leaders, scientists, and doctors are unwilling to come to grips with is that we are on the threshold of vast human annihilation. The effort to revitalize the human immune system must begin with a massive effort to return vitality and fertility to our soils.

Consider the picture painted seventy years ago by historian V. G. Simkovich in writing about the great fallen civilizations:

> Go to the ruins of ancient and rich civilizations in Asia Minor, northern Africa, or elsewhere. Look at the unpeopled valleys, at the dead and buried cities, and you can decipher there the promise and the prophecy of us. . . . Depleted of humus by constant cropping, land could no longer reward labor and support life, so the people abandoned it. Deserted, it became a desert; the light soil was washed by the rain and blown around by the shifting winds.

Perhaps the most sobering adage about history is, "The only thing we learn from history is that we learn nothing from history." As we are about to consider, this could shortly become an epitaph for our entire planet if a rapid about-face in ecological and human priorities is not made on a global scale.

Figure 2.1   Immune System of Earth at Fever Pitch

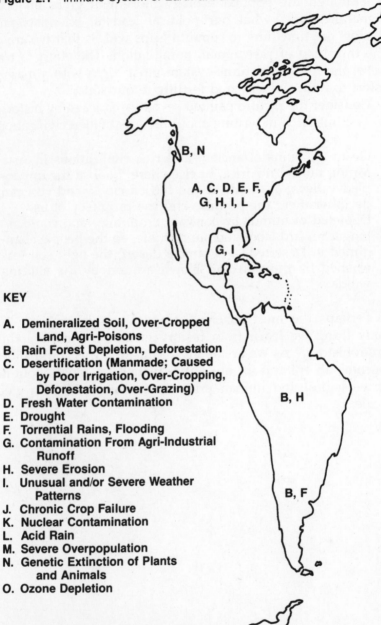

B, N

A, C, D, E, F,
G, H, I, L

G, I

B, H

B, F

O

KEY

A. **Demineralized Soil, Over-Cropped Land, Agri-Poisons**
B. **Rain Forest Depletion, Deforestation**
C. **Desertification (Manmade; Caused by Poor Irrigation, Over-Cropping, Deforestation, Over-Grazing)**
D. **Fresh Water Contamination**
E. **Drought**
F. **Torrential Rains, Flooding**
G. **Contamination From Agri-Industrial Runoff**
H. **Severe Erosion**
I. **Unusual and/or Severe Weather Patterns**
J. **Chronic Crop Failure**
K. **Nuclear Contamination**
L. **Acid Rain**
M. **Severe Overpopulation**
N. **Genetic Extinction of Plants and Animals**
O. **Ozone Depletion**

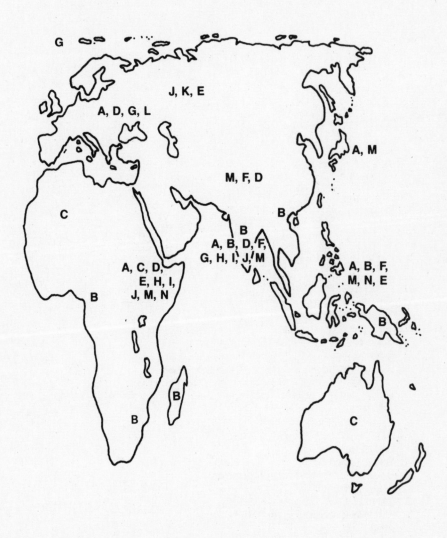

Source: *GAIA: An Atlas of Planetary Management*

3
Soil: The Living Source

No civilization has ever lived beyond the health of its soil, and only by the most artificial means have we stretched this rule and extended this civilization. The difference today is that this sword of Damocles hangs over the entire globe, rather than, as it has in the past, in a sequestered section of the globe, affecting one group of people.

Depending upon the region, unless helped by soil-building techniques (which modern farmers do not use), it takes between one hundred and one thousand years for natural forces to form one inch of topsoil. That amount can erode within a one-hour, intense thunderstorm where the land is void of dense vegetation and root systems that grow beneath it.

In the United States, combined erosion from wind and water exceeds the staggering sum of six billion tons annually. That number is increasing every year, and 1988–1989 looks to be the worst ever. Out of 100 percent of eroded soil, 90 percent is American farmland. This is dying proof that our farmers are losing their lands through destructive agricultural practices.

Good soil is 45 percent minerals, and one teaspoon of non-chemically-treated soil hosts more living creatures than there are people in the world. The European settlers found eighteen to twenty-five inches of rich topsoil in America in the sixteenth and seventeenth centuries. Stories tell of their iron plows bending and cracking on their first pass through the dense root systems. Most farmlands in the United States today are working with a mere six to nine inches of topsoil. During the autumn and spring, I have often had to slow my car to a virtual crawl going down Interstate 25 between Cheyenne, Wyoming, and Denver, Colorado, because of dense dust storms blowing like a sandblaster from West to East—Colorado farms on their way to Nebraska and Kansas.

TODAY'S "FARMER"

When I see the rather pathetic plight of American farmers, I sadly understand. They are losing their land to banks and large corporations, losing their health through toxic chemical exposure and stress; and their way of life is vanishing. In a personal sense, I feel sorry for anyone who falls on hard times, and I desire no one to suffer in a land of plenty or to lose the labor of their love, as so many of these farmers have. However, when I see the American farmer losing his land today, I believe he actually lost it a long time ago. The consequences of past acts are just coming to fruition.

The American farmer began to lose his land the first time he treated the plant instead of the soil. He lost it the first time he poisoned his land for short-term profit.

Modern agriculture has combined technology and economics to exploit the soil ecosystem for profit. The result: *modern agriculture reduces the role of soil to a substance of convenient texture that holds plants in the vertical position while chemicals are forced up their shaft. Plants stand in the field and receive a chemical enema.*

The modern farmer's approach is: *"Ah, my corn is a little wimpish this year, yellow on the leaves here. Hmm, there are aphids living on my tomatoes. Ah, there's bacteria infecting these beets."*

He then treats the disease in the plant, just like the doctor who treats only the single symptom of the patient. Modern farmers drive down to their local agricultural stores and describe the plant's symptoms to a sales person. Then they purchase chemicals recommended to suppress those symptoms.

By comparison, true farmers get out there; put their hands in the soil; smell it; let it sift through their fingers; see how it holds water; run some tests on organic matter, mineral balance, plant sugar content, and pH. They understand that the soil is the life source of the plant. They understand that the remineralization of the soil and its microbial life is paramount. They understand that the soil, not the plant, needs treatment.

A friend of mine who is an organic farmer in County Meath, Ireland, has some good advice for farmers, "Live like you won't be here tomorrow, but farm like you'll be here forever." The sacred care and trust given to the farmer is to care for the soil and, subsequently, to grow healthful food on it. This is why I say that, in a personal sense, I can feel sorry for anyone who loses their livelihood and means of caring for themselves. But our farmers lost their land long before the banks took it away. The true farmer treats the soil, just as the true physician treats the person, not the illness.

THE ROOTS OF OUR UNDERSTANDING

We can learn a great deal about the human immune system by studying the immune system of the plant, for both are ultimately dependent on the soil. No serious investigation into nutrition can be made without a thorough knowledge of the principles of soil health and its relationship to the food produced. Yet not one in a thousand nutritionists or dieticians has ever studied the soil and plant relationship.

Much of what we understand as the modern basis of good soil health and nutrition came from the great soil research pioneer, William Albrecht, Ph.D., of the University of Missouri, who published his work between 1940 and 1960. Dr. Albrecht discovered that undulant fever in livestock and humans could be cured by adding trace minerals to the soil in which their food grew. He proved that plant vulnerability to insects, fun-

gus, and disease in general were all caused by mineral deficiency and agri-chemical toxicity. Even drought resistance
came from the soil. Albrecht's work was conclusive of at least
one stubborn fact: Soil is a living substance.

During the same era, Royal Lee, D.D.S. (pictured in Figure
3.1), perhaps the world's greatest nutritionist, was integrating
Dr. Albrecht's experiments and discoveries with his own research, spanning fifty years, in plant, animal, and human nutrition. In an ever-productive career, from the early 1920s
through the mid-1960s, Dr. Lee amassed an encyclopedic
body of knowledge in plant, animal, and human health and
its links to soil, food processing, diet, and nutrition that at
every stage was forty years ahead of its time. To coordinate
and communicate nutritional breakthroughs from both his
own laboratory and laboratories throughout the world, he established the Lee Foundation for Nutritional Research, which
in its day was the world's largest clearinghouse of nutritional
information for doctors, homemakers, and agriculturalists. He
was one of that rare breed of multidisciplinary geniuses, considered by many to be the most informed food scientist of
his day.

Royal Lee was a brilliant electronic inventor. His Lee Engineering Company held more than one hundred of his electrical patents. He invented the governor motor, the Lee Flour
Mill, the Endocardiograph (heart phonocardiograph and radio frequency microphone). As a manufacturing biochemist,
Royal Lee's patents were innovative. His processing techniques remain the natural supplement industry standard long
after his patents have expired. Lee's inventions were credited
for advancing weapons control and guidance systems for the
Pentagon during World War II. His genius for simplification
of electronic design was relied on extensively by the National
Aeronautics and Space Administration (NASA) for Lunar
Guidance Systems and their motor control design.

But his first love was nutrition where his applied talents
invented and patented the cold process method for making
whole-food nutritional concentrates. This cold sterilization
technique proved to be the best method for preserving bioac-
tivity of nutrient content and is the basis of vacuum freeze
drying. Royal Lee was relentless in his passionate pursuit of

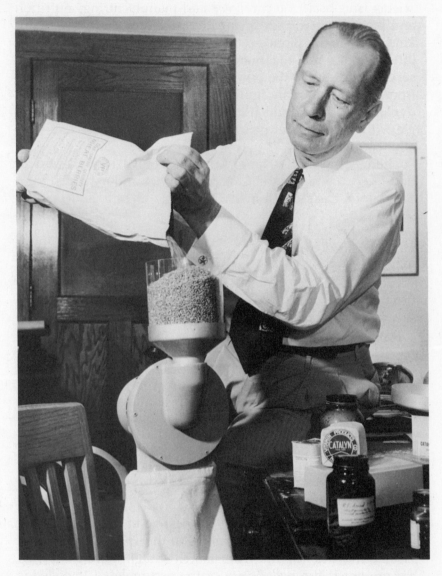

Figure 3.1 Dr. Royal Lee (1895–1967)

Perhaps the world's greatest nutritionist, Dr. Lee was also a prolific electronic inventor. Here he is working on his famous Lee Flour Mill. He designed it so the average household could have wholesome, fresh, low-heat, stone-ground flour with the vitamin-rich germ and fiber-full bran intact. His Lee Foundation for Nutritional Research was a lighthouse as food adulteration and commercialism swept the twentieth century.

science and health, technology and manufacturing, nutrition and biochemistry, and raising the quality of life for human-kind. Like many pioneers of science and philosophy, he had little patience for the manipulation of science and facts to serve and preserve the powerful vested interests that profited from the ignorance and gullibility of a trusting populace. This dynamic spirit brought him into constant conflict and strug-gle with the powerful political tools of agribusiness and food adulteration forces.

Though most of today's Americans have never heard of Royal Lee, the renowned Canadian author and naturalist John Tobe, upon Lee's death in 1967, wrote,

> Mankind has lost one of its truly great sons, with the passing of Dr. Royal Lee from this earth.
>
> I boldly state that Dr. Royal Lee did more for the health of the American people than any man living or dead. . . . I consider him one of the greatest men that America has ever produced. I say that with the full real-ization of what I am saying.
>
> He was far above any politician, far above any preacher, and he was truly America's greatest patriot, a true scientist and he was persecuted practically to death for his efforts. I know of no man, about whom I have read or heard, in my life-time who could be said to be the peer of Dr. Royal Lee.
>
> America, aye, the world, has cause to mourn the pass-ing of one of its truly great citizens. May his soul rest in peace, even though he was persecuted on earth!

To appreciate the historical perspective of the diminishing state of the human immune system in the 1990s, we must not assume that science and truth march straight ahead and that the present is the beneficiary of the accumulated knowledge of the past. Because, in many instances—and health and nu-trition is one—the past is full of deception and factual manip-ulation resulting in the inheritance of a tarnished view of scientific progress. History repeatedly proclaims that business and politics are too important to be governed by the facts of unfeigned science.

FOR DIGESTION'S SAKE, SMOKE CAMEL CIGARETTES: TO LOSE WEIGHT NATURALLY, EAT WHITE SUGAR

Following World War I, America began a demographic shift from the farm to the city. Factories lured people off the land and began packing them into large urban areas. The food supply began to change in earnest. Government food and drug regulation was increasingly serving the convenience, cost-effective, long-shelf-life demands of food processors, regardless of nutritional quality. After generations of whole and unprocessed foods, science was showing business short cuts. Within one generation the foods of commerce took over. The food supply became bleached, refined, chemically preserved, pasteurized, sterilized, homogenized, hydrogenated, artificially colored, defibered, highly sugared, highly salted, synthetically fortified (enriched), canned, and generally exposed to hundreds of new man-made chemicals. As depicted in Figure 3.2, cigarettes were advertised to aid digestion and white sugar as the modern way to lose weight.

In full-page, color advertisements in the major magazines such as *Life*, *Look*, *Newsweek*, and *Time*, R.J. Reynolds Tobacco Company ran slick ads with headlines like, *"For Digestion's Sake, Smoke Camels."* The ads featured rich and famous people claiming that Camels helped them digest food. One 1937 ad's copy said, "Scientists explain that smoking Camel cigarettes increases the flow of digestive fluids, fostering a sense of well-being and encouraging good digestion. Enjoy Camels' mildness—with meals—between meals—whenever and as often as you choose." The ad on page 38, run during the Thanksgiving season of 1937, instructed the smoker to have a Camel between each course of a five-course meal so that digestion benefitted. Copyright laws prevent duplication in this book, but in these ads cigarettes were shown to improve health. In fact, at the time, most M.D.s in the United States smoked and often recommended cigarettes to nervous patients (who were probably wired on sugar and starved of vitamins and minerals needed by the nervous system).

As the sugar ad from the 1950s displays on page 39, nutrition science and health were treated with unabashed distortion and manipulation. The ad advises weight conscious

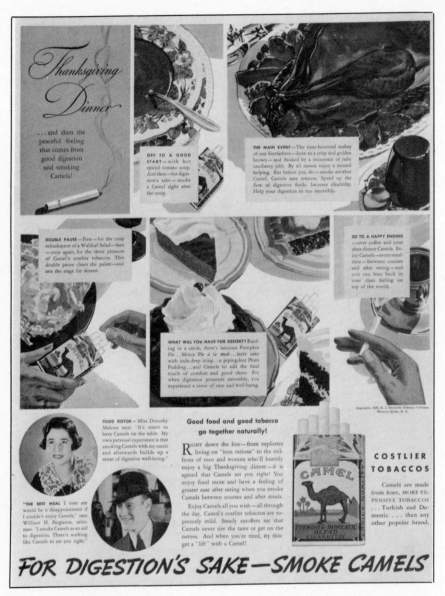

Figure 3.2 Cigarette Ad Claims That Camels Help Digest Food
c. 1937

At the same time federal courts and the FDA issued gag orders and confiscated materials of Royal Lee's writings and lectures on nutrition, ads that touted smoking cigarettes for health, like the one above, or the ludicrous one for white sugar on the facing page, met with no government opposition.

What calories are non-fattening?

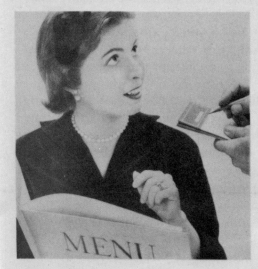

All the calories that you use up are non-fattening

The average adult uses up 2,300 to 3,200 calories a day

There are only 18 calories in a level teaspoonful of sugar

And sugar can help you cut down on the only kind of calories that can make you fat — they are the ones that come from overeating

Science shows how sugar can help keep your appetite—and weight—under control

These days, when it seems that someone is always reminding you about the calories in the things you like best, it's reassuring to remember what calories *really* are.

Calories are simply units of *energy*. All foods contain calories, but the only calories that can make you fat come from *overeating*—from over-sized portions and unneeded second helpings.

Since sugar is best known as a quick energy food, it is often singled out as a source of calories. Of course it is. But you use up as many calories as you get in a teaspoonful of sugar in just about 7½ *minutes of normal activity*.

These calories that are *spent* for energy can never be *deposited* as fat. That holds true whether the calories come from steak or apple pie, grapefruit or sugar.

Sugar is used as energy faster than *any* other food because it is absorbed into the blood stream almost immediately.

This is a helpful fact to know if you're watching your weight! That's because variations in the blood sugar level play an important role in the healthy body's appetite control system.

In clinical tests at a leading university, scientists found that people got hungry when their blood sugar level was *low*. They got hungry *more often* when they were *going* weight. But when their blood sugar level was elevated there was less sensation of hunger.

This important discovery explains why it is easier to stay satisfied on less food when you have a sweet just before a meal. It has also led to an entirely new concept of diet planning, designed to help people *cut down* on food without *cutting out* any favorite food.

These newer, more realistic diets purposely *include* sugar in foods and beverages because it makes the diet easier to get started on, easier to get used to and easier to stick to.

And if you are maintaining your present weight, isn't it good to know that sugar helps to count your calories for you?

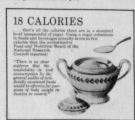

18 CALORIES

. . . that's all the calories there are in a standard level teaspoonful of sugar. Using a sugar substitute in foods and beverages actually saves so few calories that the authoritative Food and Nutrition Board of the National Research Council reported:

"There is no clear evidence that the availability in and consumption by the general public of artificially sweetened foods would be effective for purposes of body weight reduction or control."

All facts in this message apply to both beet and cane sugar

SUGAR INFORMATION, INC.
New York 5, New York

Sugar Industry Claim That Sugar is Non-Fattening
c. 1955

individuals to eat more white sugar to lose weight. Sugar, the ad scientifically explains, gives the body the kind of calorie that burns; you can't gain weight from it; therefore, sugar is good for you.

As Dr. Lee and other pioneers exposed the chronic malnutrition rampant in our nation, how indigestion was caused by the worn-out digestive tracts of the civilized diet, how dental caries, diabetes, and other diseases were caused by sugar, they were persecuted with the full power and unlimited taxpayer resources of the FDA. Dr. Lee was branded a racketeer because he promoted whole, natural, unadulterated foods with their vitamins and minerals intact. When he designed digestive aids with enzymes and calcium products to replace the loss of the minerals through processing and sugarized diets, he was branded a faddist and extremist who was duping the public. The tragedy of my parents' generation is that they grew up listening to Betty Crocker instead of Royal Lee. His work was condemned as dangerous to the public. So while Camel cigarettes and sugar were left to reap their profits, federal judges told Dr. Lee to stifle his writings and lectures, or go to jail.

We can now look back upon those days and sadly see the origins of the subversion and manipulation of the Pure Food and Drug Law by commercial interests profiting from the sale of counterfeit foodstuffs. These commercial interests have had agencies of the United States government as their front line ever since 1912, when they forced Harvey W. Wiley, M.D., from office. Pictured in Figure 3.3, Dr. Wiley was the noble founder of the United States Food and Drug Administration (FDA), then called the Bureau of Chemistry. He was also the father and architect of the nation's first Pure Food and Drug Law in 1906 (sometimes called the Wiley Act). Figures 3.4 and 3.5 illustrate the work borne of, and the reaction to, Harvey Wiley's uncompromising dedication to the truth.

Characteristic of this commercial-backed, political front line, following Dr. Wiley's removal, was Elmer M. Nelson, M.D., head of the FDA, Division of Nutrition. In testimony given in federal court to block health food manufacturers from comparing the quality of their products to ersatz counterparts, Nelson said, "It is wholly unscientific to state that a

Dr. Harvey W. Wiley (1844–1930)

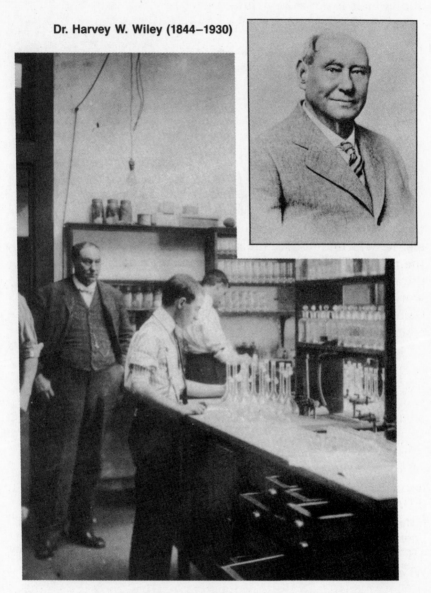

Figure 3.3 Dr. Wiley in His Laboratory

Father and architect of the nation's first Pure Food and Drug Law of 1906 (often called "The Wiley Act"), Dr. Wiley was the first chief of the Bureau of Chemistry (renamed the FDA). He fought to protect, preserve, and enhance the food supply, but was undermined by politically powerful commercial food industry forces.

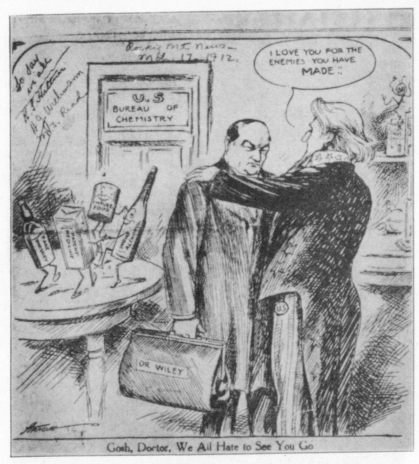

Source: *Rocky Mountain News,* c. March 1912

Figure 3.4 Cartoons Depict Reaction to Dr. Wiley's Departure From
Bureau of Chemistry

Above, as Dr. Wiley prepares to leave, on the table behind him, impure foods,
patent medicines, and ersatz substances hold hands and dance for joy. Above
right, Uncle Sam bids farewell, and laments the end of Dr. Wiley's career at
the Bureau of Chemistry.

well-fed body is more able to resist disease than a less well-
fed body. My overall opinion is that there hasn't been enough
experimentation to prove dietary deficiencies make one more
susceptible to disease." (*Washington Post,* October 26, 1949.)
This was not a mere slip of the tongue for him. Indeed, for

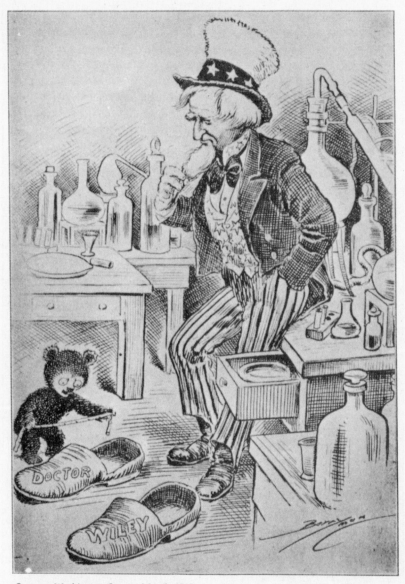

Source: *Washington Star,* c. March 1912

more than ten years, Dr. Nelson led a group of medical experts (hired mouths) to testify in courts that neither degenerative disease, infectious disease, nor functional disease could possibly result from nutritional deficiency. This, despite the landmark global studies of Dr. Weston Price ("Nutrition and

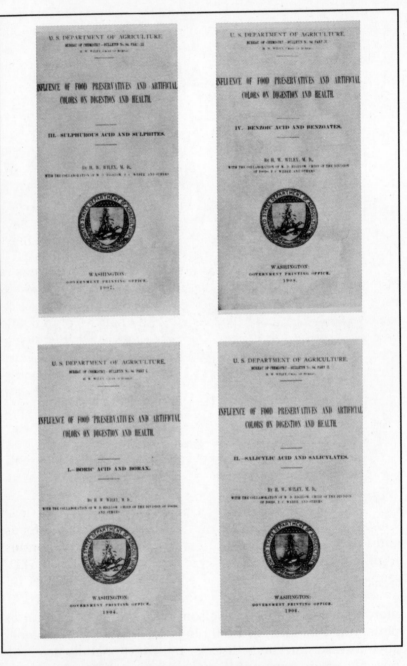

Figure 3.5 Exposing Harmful Food Additives Led to
Dr. Wiley's Undoing

Physical Degeneration," 1939); and Sir Robert McCarrison, M.D. ("Study in Deficiency Diseases"); the decades-long studies by Dr. Francis Pottenger on nutrition and tuberculosis and effects of processed, pasteurized foods on animals and humans; the great nutrient discoveries of Dr. Roger Williams at the University of Texas; and results of Dr. Agnes Fay Morgan's refined-and-enriched foods experiments at the University of California at Berkeley.

Despite literally thousands of references in scientific journals throughout Europe and North America linking nutritional status and disease, Nelson was relentless in his plan to destroy nutritional medicine. His baseless testimonies had the effect of promoting a drug approach to disease. This obscured the decades of progress that were unlocking the gates to health.

Apparently, Dr. Nelson had no respect for the warnings of his contemporary, United States Surgeon General Dr. Thomas Parran, who stated on a nationwide NBC Radio broadcast on January 18, 1941, "We have learned of the virtues of milk and of green vegetables; of fish liver oils, so rich in vitamins A and D; of the vitamin C in citrus fruits. In spite of this, every survey, by whatever method and wherever conducted, shows that malnutrition of many types is widespread and serious among the American people. We eat over-refined foods, with most of the natural values processed out of them. *Because of this, many well-to-do Americans who can eat what they like are so badly fed as to be physically inferior and mentally dull* [emphasis added]. The nutrition of the very poor is appalling." Presumably not agreeing that being "physically inferior and mentally dull" are serious conditions, Dr. Nelson and his FDA team were zealous in protecting the makers of devitalized foods, and the pharmaceutical empires, and their enormous profits, from the danger of an enlightened public. Ironically, FDA founding father Dr. Wiley had envisioned the mission of this powerful agency in reverse.

In 1929, Dr. Wiley self-published his extraordinary memoirs, entitled *The History of a Crime Against the Pure Food Law*. In prior attempts to publish conventionally, his manuscripts had mysteriously disappeared. He died within a year. His book vanished from libraries and bookshops around the nation within a matter of weeks. The Lee Foundation reprinted the book through photolithography in 1955.

Dr. Wiley's crusade to protect the health of Americans by preventing adulteration of food through refining, over-processing, and exposure to man-made chemicals makes him one of the greatest unsung heroes of the twentieth century.

Characteristic of his fearless pursuit of protecting the American public from food adulterators, he filed suit against the mighty Coca-Cola Company, to keep the artificial product from interstate transport to effectively keep the product off the market. Dr. Wiley made it clear what his vision of protecting the health of the American people was:

> "No food product in our country would have any trace of benzoic acid, sulfurous acid or sulfites or any alum or saccharin, save for medical purposes. No soft drink would contain caffeine or theobromine. No bleached flour would enter interstate commerce. Our foods and drugs would be wholly without any form of adulteration and misbranding. The health of our people would be vastly improved and the life greatly extended. The manufacturers of our food supply, and especially the millers, would devote their energies to improving the public health and promoting happiness in every home by the production of whole ground, unbolted cereal flours and meals."

One may ponder what Dr. Wiley's view would be of the purity of America's current food supply and of those charged with protecting it. What would he think of an official FDA report, "Food Defect Action Levels," recently released, that allows the following contamination of food products: A seven-ounce glass of tomato juice can contain up to twenty fly eggs (maggots); a one-pound box of macaroni can have up to nine rodent hair fragments; a one-pound box of frozen broccoli can have 276 aphids; 3.5 ounces of apple butter can have up to five whole insects; and one pound of cocoa beans can have up to ten milligrams of rodent feces.

Together, Albrecht and Lee made it clear through their studies that when we see a symptom on the plant, it will always correlate to a poison or a deficiency in the soil; when we see a disease in the human, it will relate to a poison or a deficiency in the food. This includes the previously unanticipated phenomenon of many genetically transmitted conditions, because they originated in deficiency and poisoning patterns of forebearers.

The ability of nutritional deficiencies to affect genetics via soil depletion, over-processed foods, over consumption of sugar and bad fats, and starvation was first recognized in the 1930s. In 1939, Weston Price, D.D.S., published his monumental studies on world nutrition in *Nutrition and Physical Degeneration*. Pictured in Figure 3.6, Dr. Price took his photographic sojourn to primitive cultures around the world. There, he graphically captured the racial destruction occurring as civilized counterfeit and adulterated foods found their way into the diets of indigenous people. As soon as the parents began to eat what Dr. Price called *"the foods of commerce,"* they passed along inferior genetic traits to the very next generation of offspring. Refer to Figures 3.7 through 3.11 on pages 50 through 54 for a full illustration of this phenomenon. This series is comprised exclusively of original photos taken by Dr. Price during his trips around the world. They are taken from his book and are presented here with Dr. Price's original captions.

In the conclusion to *Nutrition and Physical Degeneration*, Dr. Price wrote, "Even heredity with all its complicated nature, while in a sense immortal is itself purely physical and composed of units of proteins, minerals and vitamins called genes and in the transfer from one generation to the next must be rebuilt by the special sex cells of the parents and only by complete rebuilding can perfect hereditary traits physical and physiological, be expressed as personality and character. . . . Nature has been making normal birds, butterflies and animals for millions of years. If wild animals can do it why can not we? Is it because they, by their instinct, select the right foods and do not meddle with nature's food by changing them?"

Summarizing scientific research gathered from around the world, Dr. Lee said in 1950, "Trace mineral deficiency, it is evident, can act also to impair hereditary transmission. As these trace minerals and determinants [cell blueprints] are

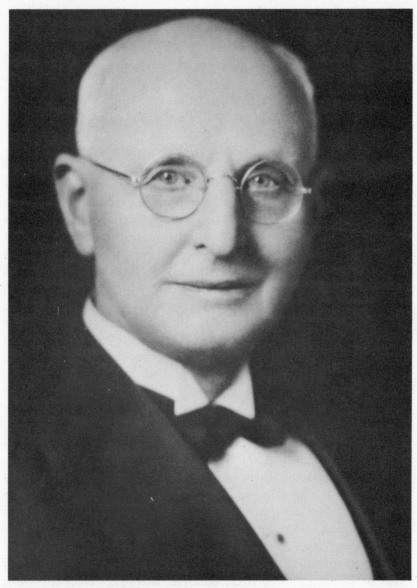

Photos and captions by permission of the Price-Pottenger Foundation, California.

Figure 3.6 Dr. Weston Price (1870–1948)

His classic book and photo journal of 1939, *Nutrition and Physical Degeneration,* documented what the refined diet of western civilization was doing to humankind around the world. The work of Dr. Price should be required reading in all schools professing any knowledge of health and disease.

combined organically into protein linkages, it is evident how the nature of these minerals in our foods are of vital importance. Compost gardening [organic gardening] in building up the organic mineral levels of the soil is here justified, and its results explained."

THE ROOTS OF OUR IMMUNITY

To begin to understand the plant's immune system and its design of resistance to disease, picture a plant growing in the soil. Along the roots of the plant grow offshoots called rootlets. Growing on the rootlets are little hair-like fungi called mycorrhiza. Mycorrhiza are fungus, yeast-type substances that are very delicate and potentially quite toxic, similar to the tiny insect that has a concentrated poison. These little fungi, mycorrhiza, secrete small amounts of highly toxic chemicals.

Mineral-rich soil is full of microbial life. It contains millions of bacteria. The primary function of this microbial life in the soil is to break down anything that falls upon the land, and to break down mineral deposits into available plant food. You might take an apple core and throw it on the land. When you come back later—if an animal hasn't yet eaten it—it's decaying. When you return still later, it's gone. The microbial life of the soil has returned it to Mother Earth, but she reclaims it in its elemental or component form. This process is called the soil cycle. By analogy, the land does not want words, it wants the alphabet. If you drop words upon the soil, it breaks down into letters. The soil wants these elemental parts in order to reconstitute them into other life forms.

This bacteria is extremely active; it is busy breaking down organic matter to release the minerals. Although bacteria suffer from constant bad press, another stubborn fact is that the overwhelming majority of bacteria are good, healthy, friendly bacteria. Why, then, doesn't this devouring bacteria attack the growing plant? The reason the plant is safe, and its roots are not attacked by the bacteria, is the *mycorrhiza*.

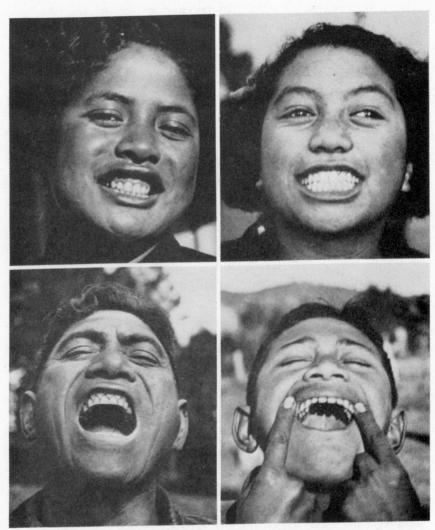

Photos and captions by permission of the Price-Pottenger Foundation, California

Figure 3.7 Since the discovery of New Zealand the primitive natives, the Maori, have had the reputation of having the finest teeth and finest bodies of any race in the world. These faces are typical. Only about one tooth per thousand teeth had been attacked by tooth decay before they came under the influence of the white man.

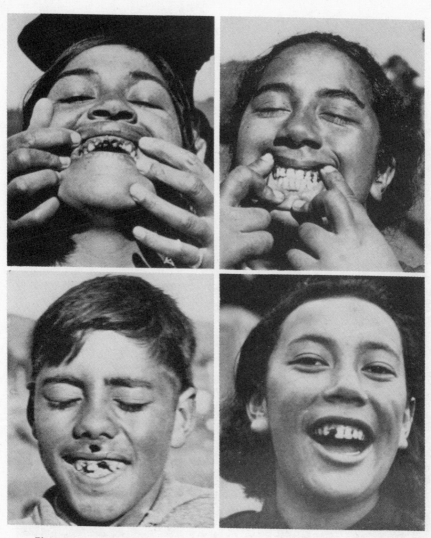

Photos and captions by permission of the Price-Pottenger Foundation, California.

Figure 3.8 With the advent of the white man in New Zealand tooth decay has become rampant. The suffering from dental caries and abscessed teeth is very great in the most modernized Maori. The boy at the lower left has a deep scar in his upper lip from an accident.

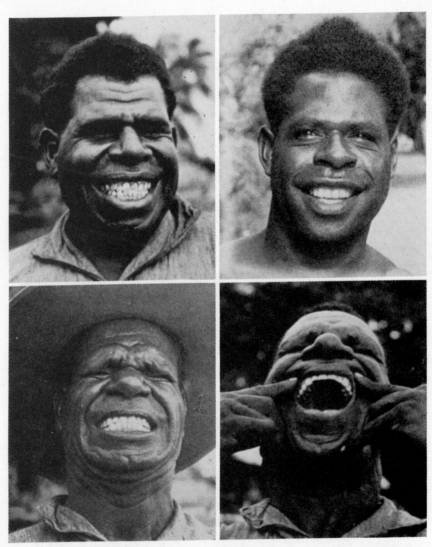

Photos and captions by permission of the Price-Pottenger Foundation, California.

Figure 3.9 Natives on the islands of the Great Barrier Reef. The dental arches here reach a high degree of excellence.

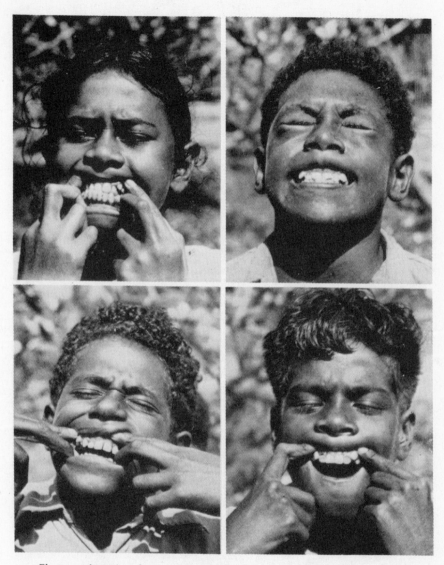

Photos and captions by permission of the Price-Pottenger Foundation, California.

Figure 3.10 The contrast between the primitive and modernized natives in facial and dental arch form is as striking here as elsewhere. These young natives were born to parents who had adopted our modern foods of commerce. Note the narrowed faces and dental arches with pinched nostrils and crowding of the teeth. Their magnificent heredity could not protect them.

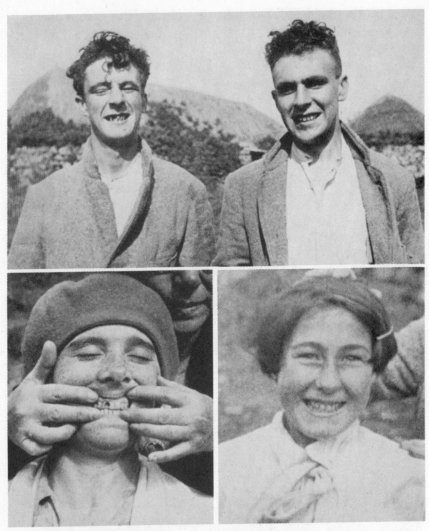

Photos and captions by permission of the Price-Pottenger Foundation, California.

Figure 3.11 Above: brothers, Isle of Harris. The younger at left uses modern food and has rampant tooth decay. Brother at right uses native food and has excellent teeth. Note narrowed face and arch of younger brother. Below: typical rampant tooth decay, modernized Gaelic. Right: typical excellent teeth of primitive Gaelic.

These mycorrhiza, living along the surface of the plant rootlets, secrete highly toxic protective substances that are anti-bacterial, called *antibiotics.* Can you think of an antibiotic that was found in a fungus? *Penicillin.* In 1929, Dr. Alexander Fleming discovered this fungal secretion when he noticed that a bacteria specimen living in a dish of culture medium had been destroyed by a spore of a mold. When the mold had matured, the surrounding bacteria had died. Fleming had discovered the *anti-biotic*, penicillin, "the wonder drug." ("Anti" means against; "biotic" means life.)

Nature gave fungi and bacteria an interesting relationship. They are natural antagonists. They keep each other in check through their competition. Each has a realm within the Earth kingdom that keeps the other in balance. Soil bacteria would otherwise attack the plant and break it down, but the plant has an immune system. The plant supports a fungus that secretes antibacterial substances that we call antibiotics.

The plant, thus protected, is free to absorb the minerals that soil microbial life has released without fear of infection from soil-borne bacteria. The bacteria and the fungus, as nature would have it, live in conflicting harmony. Not only have we found that these little mycorrhiza secrete antibiotics, but they participate in an impressively intelligent aspect of the plant, as well.

Let's say the plant needs the comparatively rare trace mineral copper, but is living in minerally imbalanced soil. Let's say there is an abundance of zinc and calcium and phosphorus in the soil, but very little copper. It has been shown repeatedly that the mycorrhiza help the plant to make an intelligent selection. These rootlet fungi help the plant to chelate, that is, bind minerals to protein for absorption. This helps them to pick up the copper. When the plant loses its mycorrhiza, it tends to get inundated by the minerals of abundance. The plant is then going to show some type of deformity or deficiency. The mycorrhiza help the plant make an intelligent selection by chelating certain of the minerals and drawing them into the sap or protoplasm of these roots and thus up into the chlorophyll, which is the "blood of the plant."

SCENARIO FOR SELF-DESTRUCTION

Nature has an excellent means of preventing inferior plant growth. Maybe a plant is, for some reason, weak, puny. Maybe it's been cut and is bleeding (plants bleed chlorophyll the way veins bleed blood). Maybe it's been damaged by a hail storm. Perhaps there was a week of 110°F days—anything you can think of that could physically injure it. Nature is a perfectionist and does not like second-rate products if she has anything to say about it.

Thus, the mycorrhiza will actually turn against and attack the plant if it is unfit for consumption. This is a protective, self-destruct mechanism. If you see a fungus growing up the stem or leaf of a plant, it is a self-produced fungus; there was something inferior about the quality of the plant. It's a self-destruct mechanism in which nothing gets wasted. Nature grows a fungus on this inferior plant, it dies, is broken down by microbial life, and begins again—until we get it right. Like a recycle center, nothing is lost; nothing is wasted. When the plant dies, only the outer form changes. The material comes back reused.

4
The Modern Approach to Agriculture

How does today's high-tech farmer deal with weak plants? The modern farmer looks down from the air-conditioned cab of his $100,000 John Deere tractor and says, "What's this?" He sees a little fungus growing on the plant and he says, "We ain't gonna put up with this. We know how to deal with the likes of you!"

He gets into his pickup truck, heads down to the agriculture chemical supply station, and returns loaded with barrels of chemosterilants, with skulls and crossbones on their labels. Now he's ready to treat the plant. In the back of his pickup truck are barrels with labels that say things like: "*Use extreme caution—do not inhale—use in well-ventilated areas—do not allow any contact with skin or hair—do not dispose of near water—keep away from livestock and feed—may cause blindness or death if taken internally—read all instructions carefully—federal law requires application in accordance with label data,*" and he thinks, "This looks good. Let's apply this to our growing food."

THE KILLING FIELDS

Remember the more than 3,500 people killed in Bhopal, India (2,000 of whom died overnight) and the two hundred thousand more who were maimed? The victims were exposed to the deadly seeping of an insecticide, *methyl isocyanate* (*MIC*). This tragedy, the worst industrial accident in world history, took place at an insecticide plant, and people were killed by a chemical that was actually meant to be sprayed on food to be consumed by animals and humans. But even this was not the largest number of human beings killed by an insecticide: *Zyklon B*, a patented German insecticide, was the instrument of Nazi genocidal psychosis used to gas millions of victims to their agonizing deaths at thirty-odd concentration camps throughout Europe from 1939 to 1945.

As a farmer applies the fungicide to the plant, it drips down the plant and descends into the soil. He returns in four or five days and the fungus is off the plant. The soil is now sterilized, no mycorrhiza. There is no more fungus on the plant, no more fungus on the rootlets, and there is nothing to prevent the bacteria from saying, "Come on, let's eat this beet."

What is the next symptom he is likely to see? The plant becomes feverish as it begins to develop bacterial infection. Plants develop infections just like human beings do when the bacterial count gets too high. The plant is now the unprotected target of all this bacteria. So the farmer's got to go back to the Ag store to get a *new* drug. This one is a complement to the fungicide. It is often applied *with* the fungicide. He sprays it on to kill the bacteria that is breaking down the plant.

He's killed the mycorrhiza, and killed the bacteria subsequently attacking the plant. Now the plant is not absorbing minerals properly and the soil is not making minerals available. The plant has lost its resistance from below. The soil ecosystem has broken down; Nature now calls upon the next line of defense, the above-ground sanitation squad—*the insects.*

"I don't want to produce second-rate products," says Mother Earth, a perfectionist. "So, if you've destroyed my first line of defense in the soil, and you're still trying to get me to produce second-rate goods, I will send aphids, I will send grasshoppers, I will send mutant bugs that you ain't never seen!"

The bugs say, "We don't care what type of drugs you put on us. We'll just mutate—because there's one thing about us insects; we don't care about bein' ugly. We don't take a long time to mutate 'cuz we don't care how we look. We just get the job done."

A LOSING STRATEGY

Modern bugs just keep on getting uglier and meaner. Sometimes I see bugs that I have never seen before in my life, in areas that I've been in many times. I look and wonder, "Where did you come from?" There is confirmation that insect species have grown, in spite of efforts to quash them. According to United States Department of Agriculture (USDA) figures, *crop loss due to insect damage has doubled since World War II, from 7 percent to 14 percent. Insecticide use is up over ten times in that same period.*

If you think this is an overstatement, consider the following. According to the World Health Organization (WHO), malaria-bearing anopheles mosquitos that are now immune to the pesticide used to control them—dichloro diphenyl trichloroethane (DDT)—have existed all over the world for many years. WHO distributes maps on which they color in certain sections of the globe where there is virtually no control of malaria, even where extraordinarily toxic concentrations of DDT are applied. These mosquitos began to develop immunity to DDT within just a few years of its agricultural introduction after World War II.

By June 1956, the WHO Executive Board issued this foreboding statement: "The conclusion was that the development of resistance to insecticides has become a serious public health problem. Thirty-two countries have reported insect resistance to DDT and other new insecticides."

Is the insect kingdom laughing at our folly? Think of it in this perspective. To equate the scale of evolution of mosquitos becoming resistant to the unimaginably toxic DDT, to put that on a human scale of evolution, would be akin to saying that so many human beings have died from bullets, human beings are now immune to being shot. You can shoot them in the chest and they're fine because so many of their species have been exposed to bullets that they mutated and are now immune to harm from bullets.

The bottom line of all this is quite simple to state and is backed by the numbers and facts: Chemosterilants (insecticides and related man-made products) do not do the job their designers envisioned them to do. In fact, they breed larger numbers of more resistant insects. They are often carcinogenic to birds, animals, and humans; destroy the soil ecosystem; and contaminate our limited supply of fresh water. They promote dependence upon a system of agriculture which is incompatible with the goal of producing healthy food.

LEADERSHIP FROM ABROAD

Recognition of these points came not a moment too soon to rescue the agricultural life of populous Indonesia. In 1989, Indonesian President Suharto, by government decree, banned at least fifty-seven organophosphate pesticides. He declared that the rice fields had become more infested with predator pests such as the rice-paddy-destroying brown plant hopper, whose natural preditors (the good guys) had been killed by all the chemicals. This is the first major producer country to take such action.

The government of Sweden, citing environmental and health concerns, has pledged to reduce pesticide use by 50 percent over five years, beginning in 1989. I think that the Swedes will find that this approach is a bit like attempting to quit smoking by cutting down.

There will always be a new bug. At a huge environmental price, we may gain a thin edge, but we'll always lose. Originally, DDT was applied to cotton for the destructive pest the boll weevil. You're not supposed to eat cotton, although now I notice people use the oil of the seeds, which are inedible.

But they soon started using DDT on food, and today when you buy Third World produce, you often get it on your tomatoes and vegetables and meat. By the time the United States Food and Drug Administration (FDA) discovers it, people will have consumed millions of tons of contamination. The United States now imports about $40 billion of food annually. Although naturalists have been laughed at for years as alarmists, this contamination was recently the page-one topic of *The Wall Street Journal*. The article reports that crop sprayers in the Third World often spray the fatal pesticide DDT, or its chemical cousins, from airplanes right onto workers in the fields. Sadly, this story was not a Third World exclusive. The National Cancer Institute (NCI) confirmed in July of 1988 what environmentalists have said for decades. After years of testing, it proved that the main chemical agent in some 1,500 pesticides—2, 4-D—is a cause of cancer in humans, particularly the American farmers who have used it enthusiastically since 1948. Sixty million pounds are applied to United States crops annually, mostly corn and wheat. In your local hardware store, it is sold under various brand names as a house and garden pesticide and weed killer. In spite of NCI's findings, the United States Environmental Protection Agency (EPA) has issued no change on the danger status of 2, 4-D.

BACKSLIDING BUREAUCRATS

In the 1950s, the slogan of the chemical industry concerning pesticides was, *"harmless to humans, but deadly to all bugs."* This, as time has proven, was profoundly wrong. Now, thanks to the efforts of lobbies funded by the powerful agricultural industry, the $7 billion pesticide manufacturers industry, and the food processing industry, all the stops have been pulled out and the pesticide barn door is open wide.

During the closing days of the Reagan Administration, the EPA responded arrestingly to the chemosterilant-food-adulteration-cancer situation. On October 11, 1988, the EPA *weakened restrictions on cancer-causing pesticides in foods*. This means the existing weak standards on the 2.7 billion pounds of pesticides used in the United States each year have been made even weaker. Three-fourths of this volume is used directly in commercial agriculture. The remaining one-fourth is used on American lawns. The EPA reports that the resulting overall balance will be better because, although the standards will be lower, they will apply to more pesticides than before.

In another example of disregard for public health, the EPA attempted to circumvent the 1958 Delaney clause of the Food, Drug, and Cosmetics Act which prohibits known cancer-causing agents in food. The EPA recently ruled to allow all foods to contain cancer-causing pesticide residues of amounts that, in the EPA's opinion, pose no more than a "negligible risk" to health. Before the EPA made these changes, only pesticides manufactured after 1972 were being regulated.

This "negligible risk" standard fails to recognize that, by definition, any exposure to a poison is too much. Poisons are cumulative. Obviously, poisons are in greater concentrated proportion to children than adults, to women than men. Often, the combination of poisons is even more deadly than the action of a poison on its own. Refer to Table 4.1 for an overview of commonly-used pesticides, the crops they're used on, and the health risks they pose.

The manipulation of numbers can also be deceiving. For instance, if they should say that *pesticide-X* may be used on avocados, and the average American eats three avocados per year, then *pesticide-X* would expose the average American to a "negligible risk." But, what if you are not the "average American" and you eat an avocado every two days, or 180 per year? You would accumulate a quantity of the cancer-causing chemical sixty times more than the EPA's unqualified "negligible risk" factor.

If the EPA's new, less-restrictive standards on pesticides should cause you to lose sleep at night, perhaps the words of FDA Commissioner Frank Young, spoken in 1988, will give you some rest: "Many seem to think we are consuming large and harmful amounts of pesticide residues. That's a myth, and another myth is that any residue, no matter how little or how legal, is harmful."

Should the EPA expect faith, trust, and respect from the American people? Have they earned it? While one might expect environmentalists to criticize the EPA as anemic, pro-industry, and foot dragging, it may come as a surprise to read

Table 4.1 Health Effects of Common Pesticides

Name	Class	Major Crop Use	Health Effects
Captan	Fungicide	Apples, peaches, almonds, seeds	Probable human carcinogen; mutagen; causes reproductive effects in animals; possible teratogen.
Daminozide	Growth Regulator	Apples, peanuts	Probable human carcinogen; causes multiple tumors at many sites in animals including the lung, liver, pancreas, nasal tissue, and vascular system; mutagen.
Mancozeb	Fungicide	Apples, onions, potatoes, tomatoes, small grains	Probable human carcinogen; mutagen; causes birth defects in experimental animals; affects kidney, thyroid, and prostate glands.
Mevinphos	Insecticide	Many fruits and vegetables	Affects nervous system; possible mutagen.
Parathion	Insecticide	Citrus, cotton, orchard crops, vegetables, fruits	Possible human carcinogen; mutagen; extremely toxic; causes nervous system effects; affects eyes in animals.
Quintozene	Fungicide	Vegetables, small grains	Probable human carcinogen; causes liver tumors in animals; possible developmental effects.

Source: Environmental Protection Agency

similar criticism in the conservative newspaper *The Wall Street Journal*. On January 20, 1989, the *Journal* described such criticisms as "justifiable," adding that the EPA often seemed "incompetent, inactive, and incoherent." It offered speculation that new laws and budget cuts were possible excuses why "EPA staffers can't do anything well." But is that truly the reason? Vermont's secretary of natural resources, Jonathan Lask, ventured further, calling former President Reagan's EPA "totally lawless." Lask said, "I've never witnessed anything like it. They just came in and totally disregarded their statutory mandates."

Surely, the EPA cannot blame the public mood for their failures. The public, who pays their wages, is in favor of environmental protection. The same *Wall Street Journal* issue confirms this: "Even the conservative Heritage Foundation, no friend to government regulation, acknowledges that Americans still tend to believe that no cost is too high to pay for environmental protection."

It would appear that modern chemical industrial science, fostered by the protective arm of the federal government, will achieve its unstated commercial goal of turning us all into cyborgs—completely dependent upon the artificial devices they will sell us. This new weaker pesticide policy will result in the release of thousands of new chemicals into our food and environment on top of the thousands already here. Incredibly, the EPA actually claims that its new "weaker but more uniform standard" will *reduce* the cancer risk. In fact, this phrase, "weaker but more uniform standard" is just typical bureaucratic jargon that means whatever they want it to mean. Under this new policy, the "negligible risk" standard could be reduced even further on raw foods if the EPA decides that the benefits to the food supply outweigh the risks. All in all, these developments force me to conclude that these are not the best days the Earth has seen.

THE FDA, THE EPA, AND INSPECTOR CLOUSEAU

In the early part of 1989, Americans were treated to a media event and public spectacle that starred the FDA and the EPA. It began when major school districts throughout the nation, afraid of exposing children to carcinogenic pesticide residues, began voluntarily to remove apples and apple products from public schools. Concurrently, an environmental group called the National Resources Defense Council (NRDC) proved that the chemical, *Alar* (*daminozide*), used to control apple ripening and appearance, is a carcinogen. Alar is a systemic chemical, which means that it is actually absorbed by the tree and flows inside the apple. Many citrus tree pesticides are systemic.

NRDC rebuked the EPA for not promptly banning Alar's use. According to NRDC, children are especially at risk from exposure. In fact, the EPA had known about this problem for years but kept calling for new tests. Under pressure they relented to take it off the market—but not for eighteen months. In the meantime, nationwide boycotts finally forced supermarket suppliers and apple growers across the nation to stop using Alar. This, in turn, ultimately led Uniroyal Inc., Alar's manufacturer, to take it off the United States market. Not an ethical decision by a long shot, Uniroyal simply acted as any profit-driven conglomerate would: by halting production of a product whose market had dried up. Typically, the EPA had nothing to do with this harmful chemical's disappearance from apples sold in the United States.

The EPA and the FDA were on the run as public outcry against them grew louder. This was highlighted by actress Meryl Streep's appearance on talk shows and her testimony before Congress imploring the nation's leaders to ban toxic agri-chemicals like Alar. It was clear that the government needed something in a hurry to show that they were on the job when it came to protecting public health. Enter Chilean grapes.

That same week, two grapes imported from Chile were found to contain traces of cyanide. Hungry for some good press, the FDA grabbed front pages across the nation by seizing all incoming Chilean fruits (thousands of tons), thereby removing them from the United States market. While TV cameras rolled, and poor Chilean farmers protested, FDA inspectors pored over tons of Chilean fruit, looking for more cyanide. They found none. But in the panic all of the fruit in warehouses, docks, and supermarkets was ordered destroyed.

This whole drama reminds me of a plot in one of the great Peter Sellers' *Pink Panther* films. In this episode, the ever-bungling Inspector Clouseau would be patrolling outside of a bank. Next to the bank, the alert inspector notices a car whose parking meter has expired. He dutifully and self-righteously begins to write a parking ticket. Meanwhile, directly behind him, an armed bank robbery is unfolding in full drama. The bad guys are running out of the bank with the money and the hostages. But Clouseau sees nothing, all the while writing up the parking ticket. Similarly, thousands of tons of imported produce full of insecticides, often those banned in this country (though manufactured here and exported), pass through our borders annually. One can't resist the feeling that this Chilean fruit episode was nothing more than an attempt to give the average consumer a false sense of security. "After all," the subliminal message asserts, "if the FDA will shut down the entire Chilean fruit industry, destroy massive quantities of their fruit at the docks, and destroy millions of dollars of fruit inventory in supermarkets because of two bad grapes, you can imagine what they would do if serious amounts of poison tried getting into this country." The big media drama accomplishes the job of giving credibility to those charged with safeguarding our health while nothing is actually accomplished. Inspector Clouseau was a comic figure of fiction; but the government's recent actions are lamentable reality. I agree with the caller to the Larry King radio talk show, who asked with sarcasm, "How could the government find two bad grapes among millions but they can't find tons of illegal drugs coming in the same way?"

Four months before this, in November 1988, *Organic Gardening* magazine hired pollster Lou Harris to check the mood of the public about organically grown and commercially grown food. Even before this Chilean episode, an overwhelming 84.2 percent of the American people said that they would buy organically grown food instead of commercially grown food contaminated with pesticides and chemical fertilizers. Another 49 percent said they would be willing to pay more money for organically grown food. After the "Chilean fruit scandal," I am sure the numbers would be even higher.

ARE THERE NO SHADES OF GRAY?

The discussion about the safety of pesticides centers on whether or not a particular chemical causes cancer. But is that the only disease worth noting? What about less grim but serious illnesses? The EPA focuses almost entirely on cancer to rule on safety. But isn't that like measuring the safety of a toy by determining only if it kills the child? What if it simply maims, blinds, or causes skin rashes? And what about the effects of *combining* pesticides? Once inside the cauldron of the human body, what are the synergistic effects of the 300-plus agricultural chemicals approved by the EPA? They don't know. No one does. But no one doubts that the answers would be frightening.

Perhaps, humans are most vulnerable to the state of the environment in the womb. Interestingly, the incidence of miscarriage has risen substantially since World War II. For this reason, a broader criterion of agricultural chemical safety should include the effects of *teratogens*—chemicals or drugs linked to birth defects, *in utero* disturbances, and spontaneous abortions. Teratogens are already known to include a variety of substances with which pregnant women are likely to be in contact. These include PCBs (polychlorinated biphenyls), mercury, lead, cigarettes, alcohol, and a broad array of common household products such as paints, cleaning agents, prescription and over-the-counter drugs, and, of course, chemical fertilizers and chemosterilants.

The Atlanta Center for Disease Control claims that 65 percent of all birth defects are of unknown etiology. Since all effects have a cause, it is fair to postulate that the vast percentage of birth defects are induced by the mother's encounters with toxic substances. Table 4.2 provides some interesting statistics from *Newsweek* magazine and the birth defects branch of the Atlanta Center for Disease Control.

For many years, the United Farm Workers (UFW) have tried to persuade Americans to boycott United-States-grown grapes because of pesticides. One of the five pesticides that the UFW is trying to ban is Captan. This particular pesticide is the one "found most frequently in residue testing on

Table 4.2   Common Modern Birth Defects

Birth Defect	Occurrence Rate per 10,000 Live Births	Description
Cardiovascular	48.0	Severe abnormalities in the structure of the heart, including the valves, blood vessels, and heart chambers.
Clubfoot	28.0	Twisted foot that does not rest properly on the ground.
Hypospadias	27.0	Misplaced opening of the penis.
Cleft Lip or Palate	15.0	Incomplete fusion of the two sides of root of mouth or upper lip.
Neural Tube	12.5	Incomplete closure of the spinal column, resulting in spina bifida—open spine; or anencephaly, a small or absent brain (always fatal).
Limb Reduction	10.0	Shortened or missing arms, legs, fingers, or toes.
Down Syndrome	9.5	Also called mongolism. Often characterized by mental retardation and various physical defects.

grapes" according to environmental disease expert Dr. Marion Moses. Captan is structurally similar to *thalidomide*, the sedative blamed as the agent that caused thousands of infants to be born without legs or arms in the early 1960s. Statistics recently researched by Dr. David Schwartz of the University of Washington, and reported in the *American Journal of Public*

Health, revealed that women living in California farm counties where pesticides are freely used were 190 percent more likely than California women in non-farming counties to have babies with significant birth defects such as limb reductions and other deformities. It is no wonder that the first words of any mother, when her baby is born, are invariably, "Is my baby normal?"

The United Nations estimates that our planet is subjected to two million tons of pesticide applications every year. (A ton equals two thousand pounds.) At a rate of 20 million tons per decade, how can any rational argument be made that, when safely applied, they pose no threat?

THE CARCINOGENIC CORN CROP OF 1988

The severe summer drought of 1988 has underscored the man-made weakness in our American soils caused by dependence on artificial chemicals. The smallest corn harvest since 1970 was also the largest toxic harvest of the cancer-causing, fungus-produced *aflatoxin*. The fungus is called *Aspergillus flavus*. Aflatoxin is so poisonous, it is reported to be 100 times more capable of causing a cancer than the notorious industrial pollutant PCB. The inferior corn crop was unable to resist this fungus-based carcinogen. So significant is this agricultural disaster that *The Wall Street Journal* featured it as the front page leading story on February 23, 1989, giving it an unheard-of four pages of coverage. The front page headline declared: "Spreading Poison; Fungus in Corn Crop, A Potent Carcinogen, Invades Food Supplies; Regulators Fail to Stop Sales of Last Fall's Harvest Laden With Aflatoxin." The first sentence could well serve as a foundation for an overhaul of the agricultural practices of our country: "OQUAWKA, ILL.— From the corn fields that stretch for hundreds of miles around this Mississippi (river) town, one of the most potent cancer-causing agents known to science is coursing into the nation's food supply."

This is a textbook case-in-point of a soil-based weakness transmitted to the vulnerable hybrid plant. According to *Time* magazine, at least nine states have confirmed the aflatoxin corn contamination. To dilute corn, brokers are mixing the previous year's stored corn crop with the unfit harvest of 1988. In response to this toxic problem, the FDA is protecting the farmers by raising the permissible level of aflatoxin contamination on corn in interstate commerce by 1,500 percent! Is our nation's "bread basket" becoming a "dead basket"? In the past, this corn would have been condemned as "unfit for human or animal consumption" and destroyed. Asians and Africans exposed to aflatoxin have the world's highest rate of liver cancer. But today, with the financial pressures overriding all other concerns, the solution chosen is to just lower the standard. When it comes to business-versus-health, it's politics as usual.

The United States Midwest produces about a third of the world's corn crop and it is the most important commodity produced in Iowa, Illinois, and Indiana. As much as 36 percent of the tested corn in some Midwestern states shows positive for aflatoxin. Hundreds of thousands of pounds of milk have had to be destroyed from Texas to Wisconsin, from Minnesota to Florida. Japan and the Soviet Union are rejecting United States corn products and bulk shipment, unless it is certified to be exclusively 1987 harvest. Corn-laden ships in New Orleans have been offloaded.

Blaming the drought for the aflatoxin contamination is a bit like blaming a smoker for the great Chicago fire. The prevailing conditions had to be right for the ignition.

CAUSE: MODERN FERTILIZER

To try and decipher the natural cause of this aflatoxin tragedy, I contacted Lee Fryer, a nationally respected natural farming expert who has studied, created, and written about soil health and fertility for more than thirty years. According to Mr. Fryer, half of the petro-type nitrogen fertilizer sold in the United States is applied as anhydrous ammonia (83 percent N) or as ammonia solutions (aqueous ammonia). He said, for the record, that the aflatoxin infestation is a direct—and anticipated—result of using this type of ammonia fertilizer and not replenishing the soil.

"They won't have any aflatoxin once they balance the nutrition of the crop," he said. "Straight ammonia and nitrogen destroys the humus in the soil." As soil vitality declines, the stress imposed by a drought such as the one in 1988 is only a catalyst to reveal the soil's inherent susceptibility, as Figure 4.1 shows. As we discussed earlier, nature will take over to destroy deficient produce.

BLOWING IN THE WIND

What would you think of a paper products company whose various paper goods were all stored unwrapped in a large warehouse? If the owner left all the windows and doors wide open one day and a fierce wind, like a thief in the night, blew all the paper goods away, wouldn't you criticize the owner for then going to the federal government and asking for disaster aid to cover the losses that he claimed were "due to natural forces?" Yet, this is essentially what is occurring right now to the remaining precious topsoil on countless millions of acres throughout the farm regions of the American West and Midwest. Farmers want federal aid to replace soil they lost through neglect. We don't need Woodie Guthrie songs and Henry Fonda movies to recall the Dust Bowl of the 1930s. For it is alive and well in America's farmland today.

North Dakota in these last years of the twentieth century is a current version of the worst Great Plains Dust Bowl scenes imaginable. In 1988 alone, the state lost 3.5 million acres of soil to the wind. The little town of Linton was reported to have lost five inches of topsoil in the past year, leaving only sterile subsoil behind. The state as a whole lost its wheat crop and 60 percent of its corn as a direct result of wind erosion. Anyone visiting this ravaged area can see for themselves that only lifeless subsoil remains.

The Soil Conservation Service (SCS) of the United States Department of Agriculture (USDA) estimates that at least eight million more acres will be endangered in the coming years. In news reports, university conservationists have said that that number is too low and could actually be closer to fourteen million acres.

Anyone who has ever worn a hat in North Dakota between November and May, the windiest time of year, knows that twelve-mile-per-hour wind is a mere breeze. Yet, the parched

How Aflatoxin Invades the Corn Plant...
and Where the Crop Goes

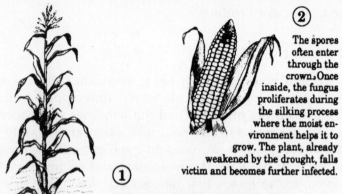

② The spores often enter through the crown. Once inside, the fungus proliferates during the silking process where the moist environment helps it to grow. The plant, already weakened by the drought, falls victim and becomes further infected.

① Under extremely dry conditions like the Midwest experienced last summer, with day-time highs of about 100 degrees and evenings in the upper 70s, the soil-borne fungus (Aspergillus flavus) becomes dust-like and airborne.

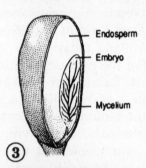

Endosperm

Embryo

Mycelium

③ As the kernel reaches maturity, the fungus moves through the base of the grain and branches into the embryo in the form of hair-like mycelia. The largest accumulation of toxin occurs during this stage. Following the harvest, mycelia can continue growing in damp and unaerated storage bins.

Supply and distribution for crop year 1987-1988*
(In millions of bushels)

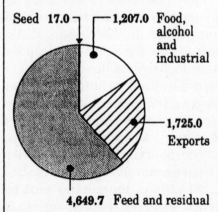

Seed 17.0 — 1,207.0 Food, alcohol and industrial

1,725.0 Exports

4,649.7 Feed and residual

*Preliminary figures; September 1987 - August 1988
Source: U.S. Department of Agriculture

Figure 4.1 Effects of Aflatoxin

North Dakota topsoil is so exposed and fragile from lack of rain, that a mere twelve-mile-per-hour wind creates havoc with the soil. As a result of severe soil erosion, *Acres USA* reports that some of North Dakota's communities are on the verge of becoming ghost towns.

SCS admits that the neighboring states of Wyoming and Montana have suffered more than at any time since they began keeping records in 1955. SCS says that at least twenty-three million acres are "in condition to blow" in the immediate future.

Again, the drought of 1988 surfaces as the last straw that topples a system of agriculture that does not treat nature as a full partner. The Great Plains, bread basket of the world, lies parched and bare. Gone are its native grasses and vegetation that anchor the soil. Vital to hold the soil, stabilize the water table, and halt the wind from stripping exposed land, trees have been removed to allow the large soil-compacting farm machinery easier movement in the fields and planting from horizon to horizon.

In the 1930s, dust storms created by wind erosion were so fierce that ships in the Atlantic Ocean became covered with soil blown by the jet streams from the Midwest. Congressmen would open their windows in Washington, D.C., to find Kansas topsoil dirtying their desks. We are close to returning to those days.

In the 1987–1988 pre-drought season, about 12 million acres, or 19,000 square miles (an area the size of Massachusetts and Maryland combined), were severely eroded by wind. But since the drought of the summer of 1988, estimates closer to the 25-million-acre figure are commonly heard. For the sake of comparison, SCS records show that in 1977, less than 5 million acres, still too high, were eroded by wind. Kansas Congressman Dan Glickman stated in March of 1989, "It's no secret the central part of America is blowing away right now." The states suffering the worst wind erosion are Colorado, Wyoming, Montana, Nebraska, New Mexico, North Dakota, South Dakota, Kansas, Oklahoma, and Texas. Clearly, North Dakota heads the list, followed by Texas. All of these states boast agricultural land grant colleges. Since the lessons of the 1930s are there for the learning, we should each draw our own conclusions.

MY FIRST ENCOUNTER: THE MISSISSIPPI DELTA

My first trepidation about this whole agricultural predicament began more than a decade ago. In 1972, while lost driving on some back roads in south-central Mississippi, I was attracted by a large fire on a harvested corn field. I stopped to ask a farmer directions. Then I asked why he was burning the remains of his field rather than turning the tailings under to create richer soil. He frowned as he told me that the soil was sterilized through years of chemosterilant applications and that there was not enough microbial life remaining in the soil to break down the fiber before the next spring planting. Incredible as it seemed, this once-fertile soil was now incapable of even rotting and composting. The farmer acknowledged that the lack of worms in the soil was proof of how sick it was.

The place about which I write had been one of the most naturally God-blessed regions on Earth, the Mississippi Delta. Ten thousand years ago, the glaciers receded and cut a huge delta. As the glaciers pressed forward and, then, backward, they left the pulverized, crushed, mineral-rich rock dust of mountains behind. This created a fertile, minerally abundant soil, constantly replenished by the silt washed onto it by the ever-flooding Mississippi River. Pioneering farmers, who moved westward to claim their piece of this soil, built empires and fortunes shipping abundant crops to a growing nation and the world by way of the Mississippi River.

But after 200 years of cropping the land, building levies along the river to prevent flooding (which would return minerals from the riverbed to the topsoil), and never adding minerals back in, the land was exhausted and nearly vanquished by the 1920s. This was just at the time when the United States chemical fertilizer industry began.

THE ORIGIN OF CHEMICAL AGRICULTURE

The agri-chemical industry, which utilizes chemicals, not natural methods, in agriculture, was born out of a paper presented in the 1840s to the British Royal Academy of Sciences by a renowned German chemist. Baron Justus von Liebig, who in 1831 invented the anesthetic *chloroform*, now analyzed human and plant ash and determined that nitrogen, phosphorus, and potassium (NPK) were all the minerals plants needed. If fed synthetically to plants, he reasoned, farmers could force plants to grow and support healthy humans. In 1855, Liebig published *Agricultural Chemistry*. This book became the founding testament for the German chemical industry (the richest in the world today), through which they began aggressively to market the NPK idea to farmers. The industry suppressed all opposition to their *"artificial manure,"* as it was then called. As a result, it flourished in Germany and was soon exported around the world. Had Liebig known about trace minerals, fungus, and microbial life, he would have undoubtedly realized what a deadly new science he was launching.

Despite his widespread success and fame, Liebig, a talented chemist, began over time to discern his error, though too late. In one of his last works, *The Natural Laws of Husbandry*, Liebig reversed his advocacy of man-made manipulation of the land and wrote, "Nature herself . . . points out to man the proper course of proceeding for keeping up the productiveness of the land." At the end of his life, in 1873, Liebig expressed deep remorse for his misguided contribution, wishing it had never been offered. His latter revelation is duly recorded in the 1899 edition of the *Encyclopaedia Britannica*.

Some twenty years after Liebig's death, famed German naturalist Julius Hensel published a short book called *Bread From Stones*. In it he exposed as "nonsense" the "artificial manure," or NPK theory, and instead encouraged farmers to spread a finely crushed, minerally rich *rock dust* on their land to remineralize their overworked soil. Those who did were amazed at the quality, strength, and drought resistance of their crops.

But the thriving German chemical industry launched a vicious campaign to discredit Hensel and promote their hero and golden goose, Liebig. The German chemical industry either published or controlled most of the agriculture journals of the day, which, as today, accounted for the vast percentage of their advertising revenues, and used them to advance their artificial products and squelch all arguments for natural alternatives. Soon after it was published, one could not find Hensel's book with a search warrant. Although his rock dust theory never became popular, the soil's need for minerals to sustain microbial life and build strong plants that were full of mineral-dependent enzymes never changed. An unaccepted fact is a fact nonetheless.

In the midst of a mindset of chemical weed eaters and pest killers, nature managed to produce a few odd men and women within whom the natural design could be discerned and taught. One such teacher of nature was Sir Albert Howard, the modern-day founding father of the natural agriculture renaissance. Sir Howard was an Englishman, mentor to American naturalist J. I. Rodale, who went on to create the Rodale natural farming and foods publishing empire.

In 1940, Oxford University published Howard's greatest work on natural farming, entitled *An Agricultural Testament*. In this book, Howard supported Hensel's rock dust theories and addressed the misguided origins of chemical farming. "The principle followed, based on the Liebig tradition, is that any deficiencies in the soil can be made up by the addition of suitable chemicals [made-made]," he wrote. "This is based on a complete misconception of plant nutrition. It is superficial and fundamentally unsound. It takes no account of the life of the soil, including mycorrhizal association—the living fungus bridge which connects the soil and sap. Artificial manures lead inevitably to artificial nutrition, artificial food, artificial animals, and finally, to artificial men and women."

ARTIFICIAL FERTILIZER EFFECT ON PLANT NUTRITION

Thanks to what the chemical agriculture industry calls "artificial manure," supermarket produce appears to be giving today's Americans more salt and less nutrition than generally recognized. In the spring of 1989, Nutrient Testing Laboratories, Ltd. (NTL), of Babylon, New York, ran mineral analysis tests on commercial produce from various regions around the United States. The results clearly showed dissimilarity in nutrient content according to soils of different regions. Sodium levels, reflecting artificial fertilizer use, were particularly high in all the commercially grown produce tested.

Using a "wet ash" method, NTL, an independent testing lab, measured the mineral content of apples, broccoli, carrots, celery, green peppers, peas, potatoes, red beets, spinach, string beans, and tomatoes purchased from supermarkets in five states: California, Colorado, Florida, Massachusetts, and New York. Where the food was grown was noted. Their test was designed to uncover mineral imbalance in the soil on which these foods are grown.

First, NTL analyzed the foods for their content of thirteen minerals: aluminum, boron, calcium, copper, iron, magnesium, manganese, molybdenum, nitrogen, phosphorus, potassium, sodium, and zinc. Then, they compared parts per million per 3.5 ounce raw portion for each of the eleven foods. Based on this data, NTL reported that mineral content in each food category tested varied widely from region to region. For example, there was three times more phosphorus in California potatoes compared with New York samples. Florida's tomatoes had eighteen times more calcium than samples from Massachusetts.

While some foods contained *no* amounts of certain important trace minerals such as boron and zinc, all eleven foods tested contained high levels of sodium. To compare this to changes over time, NTL used the famous H. J. Heinz Nutrition Chart of 1949. As a result, NTL discovered that the sodium content of each food tested has increased substantially during the last forty years. This recent elevation in sodium, NTL reports, is likely caused by commercial produce farmers' dependence on inorganic fertilizers. These "artificial manures" are highly concentrated sources of inorganic salts.

The rise in sodium is just one illustration of how plants receive only what they are given by their care givers. Rather than well-balanced soil, full of myriad trace elements and minerals, modern soils are cauldrons of inorganic chemicals made and mixed by chemical companies and fictitiously called "plant food." Business practices being what they are, the amounts and ingredients of inorganic fertilizer can vary widely, contingent upon supply, demand, profit, and economic conditions. This, in turn, contributes to the disparity of nutrient content from region to region and, most likely, from farm to farm.

These findings are significant to those who would hope to balance their personal body chemistry by eating various foods that they assume are also balanced. For instance, NTL found that Colorado's spinach had five times more iron than Florida's sample. Based on this data, iron-deficient Floridians doctoring themselves with store-bought spinach may have disappointing results.

Although NTL research is based only upon a short-term study, certain of their conclusions cannot be ignored. Their tests prove that, in 1989, food is not minerally consistent from one region to the next, a direct reflection of soil quality and depletion. It underlines the fact that artificial fertilizers change the potential nutritional value of fruits and vegetables that most American's eat.

The conclusions of the NTL study come as no surprise to organic growers long familiar with the "nutrient quality" issue in produce. The United States government was warned of this over fifty years ago in sworn testimony by their own people. Here is one graphic example of such testimony before a select Senate Committee by Morris L. Cook, an engineer of the United States National Resource Board, in 1936.

Our country is afflicted with earth disease . . . as the matter now stands, and with continuance of the manner in which soil is now being squandered, this country of ours has less than 100 years of virile national existence. If that represents a reasonably accurate statement, it is vastly more significant that we have probably less than twenty years in which to build up the technique [soil building] . . . and most difficult of all, to change the attitude of millions of people who hold that ownership of land carries with it the right to mistreat and even destroy their land, regardless of the effect on the total national state.

While he was head of the Bureau of Chemistry, Dr. Wiley created a Soil Department, which hired trains to deliver soil samples from every county in the United States and used them in greenhouse growing studies conducted outside of Washington, D.C. Dr. Wiley considered the health of the soil to be an inseparable issue of food quality and therefore instituted a huge research project to help increase soil fertility throughout America. Upon his removal from office in 1912, the project was abandoned.

ENZYMES: SPARK PLUGS OF LIFE

As mentioned in the previous section, the health of the soil's microbial life depends upon the minerals in the soil, and so does the most important ingredient in plant, animal, and human biochemistry: the enzyme. An enzyme is a large protein molecule, containing vitamins, amino acids, and trace minerals such as zinc, selenium, manganese, and copper. All metabolic processes at every level of the cell depend upon the life-sustaining action of enzymes. Without their transforming catalytic action, life processes slow down until, when enzyme activity is too low, life is no longer sustainable in a physical form. This is how many chemical weapons, such as "nerve" gas, can kill. Though outlawed by international treaty (but often ignored as recently seen in the Middle East countries of Iraq and Iran), nerve gases destroy their victims by inhibiting enzyme activity. Demineralization of the soil and mere chemical NPK application has left the vast majority of crop land deficient in the trace minerals needed to manufacture enzymes in the plant and higher species that consume them. First plants, then animals, then humans suffer.

No species can utilize ingested substances without enzymes. The processing, refining, pasteurizing, and finally cooking of foods all contribute to enzyme destruction. In fact, milk is declared pasteurized when the chemist finds no enzymes present in the milk. This places intense demand on our own organs such as the liver and pancreas to manufacture enzymes, because the food is not supplying them.

Even so, the body must have a store of the enzyme-building materials such as trace minerals, amino acids, and vitamins in order to manufacture enzymes. Often, the enzymes vital to the human immune system need the rarest trace minerals as components. Enzyme physiology can be likened to super computers, where potency and size are unrelated. A microchip speeds along powerful functions just as the rarest trace mineral transforms an enzyme into a critical catalyst, releasing tremendous energy.

Hormones, the secretions of endocrine glands, are the biochemical masters of the human body. They are formed from trace elements and vitamins such as iodine and vitamin E contained in and made available by enzymes. For example, the thyroid must have sufficient quantity and quality of the trace element iodine to form the hormone thyroxine. The pancreas requires trace minerals chromium and zinc to make insulin, the hormone that controls blood sugar. The sex steroid hormones of the gonads require vitamin E and fat-soluble vitamin factors as precursors. Manganese and vitamin E are vital to pituitary hormone production, while vitamin D is very similar to the calcium-controlling parathyroid hormone.

Edward A. Johnston, M.D., writing in *The Journal of the American College of Proctology*, stated: "All the ductless glands [endocrine glands] must have one or more of the vitamins in order to secrete their vital fluids [hormones], and, if deprived of the vitamins, will atrophy and cease to function."

One has only to be clear on one essential fact to understand how important minerals in the soil are to the human form. That fact, simply stated, is: Plants do not manufacture minerals; they absorb them. From where shall they absorb them, and from where shall human beings obtain the right form of minerals and enzyme materials?

SUSTAINABLE APPROACHES TO AGRICULTURE

For those experienced with natural farming methods, there are some outstanding and advanced techniques available. All of the following are suitable for restoring soil health. The Bio-Dynamic Method, as demonstrated in Australia, is one of the most sophisticated topsoil builders there is. For the purpose of this consideration, however, our first objective is to apply first aid and rescue techniques to reverse centuries of soil abuse. Outlined here are four proven methods to quickly remineralize the soil and regenerate microbial life.

They are synergistic together as well as effective independently.

1. Seaweed fertilizer and seaweed folier sprays. The ocean is the perfect epicenter of planetary nutrition and source of a vast spectrum of trace minerals. All ocean products are imbued with minerals. American school children are taught that the Indians on Cape Cod showed the Pilgrims how to plant corn by placing fish heads in the rows for fertilizer. While we can and do pollute the sea, we have not yet depleted the sea of its mineral wealth. Trillions of tons of every known and unknown trace mineral reside in seaweeds, fish emulsions, kelp, and other harvest of sea forms. Since the seas have covered all the land at different stages in history, no mineral form has escaped merging with the sea. I am not aware of a single mineral or element of our planet not found in the oceans. While the soil can be nourished with the spreading of seaweed, even more rapid plant health can be obtained by folier spraying of finely powdered seaweed directly on the growing plant and tree. Trace elements such as iodine are rarely found in inland crops, but can be part of a healthy plant thousands of miles from the sea through folier sprays. The tiny trace minerals can absorb directly into the leaf, and many insects are repelled by it. I have twenty plum trees that have never produced bad fruit and never suffer insect damage. They were raised exclusively on folier seaweed sprays (1,200 miles from the nearest ocean).

While the soil is being rebuilt, seaweed sprays are like a blood transfusion to the crop or tree. Seaweed fertilizers have four major advantages over synthetic petro-chemicals: their cost is relatively miniscule, the supply is nearly inexhaustible, they are non-toxic and non-polluting, and they build resistant healthy plants.

2. Finely ground rock, known as "rock dust" or "stone meal." I know of no method more capable of rapid remineralization of our crop lands, pastures, and forests than the "rock dust" method. This concept of grinding rock into a fine powder to dust upon the soil was developed in Germany by Julius Hensel in the 1890s. Dr. Albrecht, Dr. Lee, and organic farming advocate and famed publisher J. I. Rodale all encouraged the use of rock dust to remineralize soil.

It seems certain that the healthiest people on the planet Earth, the Hunzas, living in the Karakorum Range in the Himalayas, situated between Pakistan, Afghanistan, China, and the Soviet Union, to a large degree owe their fabled vitality and unequaled longevity to rock dust. They live at an elevation of 8,400 feet, surrounded by 25,000-foot peaks and the vast Ultar Glacier, from which they receive their water for drinking and irrigation. They are the living paradigm of organic farming and agriculture. Sir Albert Howard, in his book, *An Agricultural Testament*, wrote glowingly of the Hunzas, their agriculture, and their use of rock dust. Howard explained, "The staircase cultivation of these hillmen receives annual dressings of fresh rock-powder, produced by the grinding effect of the glacier on the rocks and carried to the fields in the irrigation water."

Another Englishman, G. T. Wrench, M.D., in his wonderful 1938 book, *The Wheel of Life*, reported extensively on his studies concerning the cause of rampant health among the Hunza people and wrote of their annual renewal of the soil by "a sprinkling of black glacier-ground sand." He noted that the crushed rock "plant food" kept the fruit trees, vegetables, and grains virtually free of any disease. The cherished apricot trees of the Hunza yielded nutritious fruit for a hundred years, whereas the common life span of such a tree in the United States is about twenty-five years. They call their water "glacial milk."

American farmers, with all their expensive industrial resources, have overlooked this simple proven method for retaining the mineral health of plants and of soil fertility. Though a humble Kentucky farmer named Albert Carter Savage published his life experiences using rock dust in 1942 in a pamphlet called "Mineralization," I would wager that not one in 100,000 American farmers has ever heard of rock dust. On his title page, Savage wrote, *"Will it reach you in time?"*

The nations of Austria, Switzerland, and Australia have small rock dust industries, and their supporters are zealous in documenting the wonderful results they obtain. Results are apparent within a few months, while soil microbial life vastly increases within only weeks. Small experimental areas using rock dust in the Austrian forests have produced inspiring results in an ancient but dying forest. Glacial rock and gravel, or mixtures of non-glacial rocks containing a wide range of minerals, pulverized into a powder and spread upon the land at a rate of three or four tons per acre, will quickly remineralize the soil. This is necessary because microbial life must be supported with minerals to assist in the mineral absorption into the plant.

The finest study and theoretical discussion of rock dust and its global potential can be found in the monumental work by John D. Hamaker, *The Survival of Civilization*. In this 1982 book, Hamaker accurately predicted the massive forest fires of 1987 and 1988, which were the worst in recorded history. Even as I write, 3.5 million acres of Yellowstone National Park in Wyoming and Montana are burning to death. These fires, in turn, release even more stored carbon from the land into the air in the form of carbon dioxide (CO_2), accelerating the Greenhouse process, which we discuss in detail in Chapter Five. As those forests burn and global deforestation continues (tropical rain forests equal to the size of France are cut down each year), there are fewer trees to inhale the carbon dioxide from the air and exhale oxygen (O_2) into the air. Green life constitutes the lungs of this planet, and our lungs are shrinking; being surgically removed, bulldozed, and burned. Airplanes currently dropping chemical fire retardants over burning forests could be better used to drop tree and plant-stimulating rock dust over existing forests to remineralize their soils. Rock dust may well be the key to saving and restoring the agricultural capacity of our planet.

3. Colloidal soft rock phosphate. Do not confuse colloidal soft rock phosphate with common hard phosphate rock, which is not readily soluble in water and therefore less available to the plant. The advanced soil work of Dr. Carey Reams, in Orlando, Florida, from the late 1920s through the early 1980s, promotes the electrical properties in soil to activate release of the elements. I have seen sticky clay soils transformed into loose, healthy soil within one year of a one-ton-per-acre application of colloidal soft rock phosphate. This substance comes from non-limestone, ocean vertebrate deposits in the Earth. In one ton of this essence of fish bone meal, there are sixty pounds of compound colloidal phosphate. It acts more as a soil catalyst than a fertilizer.

One of the most unusual properties of colloidal soft rock phosphate is that it keeps minerals, such as calcium, near the top of the soil and prevents minerals from gravitating too deep for plant roots to reach. It tends to "float" in the soil, like dust in the air, and moves upward, thus catching and returning minerals to the surface. It retards erosion, increases water retention, prevents soil from blowing away, loosens soil, improves tilth, feeds the healthy bacteria, and provides essential phosphorus.

Its presence in soil will increase the natural flavor of fruits and vegetables because of the increased mineral content. The higher the mineral content in the plant, the more resistant it is to insects and drought. The higher mineral content also causes a higher levulose (natural fruit sugar) content.

The higher the levulose content, the lower the freezing point of the plant. Because water freezes first, the higher mineral and levulose content retards freezing due to lower water weight in the plant. A plant deficient in minerals and levulose, but full of water, is very susceptible to frost damage. A highly mineralized plant can thaw out and still be in good shape. In 1962 and 1963, almost half of all the groves in Florida were permanently ruined by unexpected killer frosts. By comparison, in Florida, citrus grove soils treated with soft rock phosphate showed vastly superior resistance to frost. Those groves in Dr. Reams' care never suffered a single casualty, and still stand bearing good fruit to this day.

Agricultural state land grant colleges, whose livelihoods depend upon large chemical company research grants, have virtually ignored Dr. Ream's lifetime of landmark research and development.

4. Composted organic matter. Soil life depends upon the presence of microorganisms and minerals. Without microorganisms, minerals might just as well be sealed in a tomb as far as a plant is concerned. A constant renewing of the microorganisms by the addition of compost would significantly increase the rate of creation of topsoil.

As our connection with life on the Earth is topsoil, how can one overstate this point? The preservation of topsoil by recycling organic waste from foodstuffs, bones, and residual materials from harvests would immeasurably add to the topsoil.

5

The Atmospheric Immune System

Let's leave the soil and head for the sky. High above the land are majestic layers of atmosphere. Of particular importance is the ozone layer. It is miles above the planet, keeping the solar ultraviolet (UV) radiation in balance. Today, we see gaping holes developing in the ozone layer. Like the tragic effects of man-made chemicals on the soil, it is again the man-made chemicals that have unexpectedly sailed off into space damaging the ozone layer.

OZONE DESTRUCTION

Chlorofluorocarbon (CFC), a refrigerant sold under the name of *freon*, is the main chemical culprit. It rises into the stratosphere where it reacts with UV radiation from the sun. This breaks up the CFC, releasing two halogen molecules, chlorine (an oxidizing agent), and bromine, molecules that destroy the

UV-filtering ozone layer. If we stopped emitting this substance today, it would take about 100 years to regenerate the ozone layer.

Through our own actions, just as our own abuse of the soil has rendered us disease-pregnable, we have torn holes in the ozone layer. We have ripped the fabric of the immune system of the atmosphere, and scientists are predicting that, as a result, many millions of cases of skin cancer as well as severe temperature changes will occur. One of the most sobering facts of this ozone depletion is that no one, not one scientist in the world, ever predicted this phenomenon. Because of this, it is reasonable to assume that many other environmental time bombs ticking throughout the planet will make sudden unpredicted appearances. Meteorologists have been as accurate as stockbrokers in forecasting what has been popularly called the "Greenhouse Effect," as we will learn later in this chapter.

The United States banned the use of CFC as an aerosol propellent in spray cans back in 1978. But the degree of the ozone depletion problem has not been thoroughly understood until recently. The increased UV penetration from the sun's rays augers ill for all plant and animal life.

FREE RADICALS

Plants constantly exposed to unfiltered sunlight may severely suffer through a potentially destructive process called "free radical activity." A free radical is a molecule that has an unpaired electron in its orbit. As such, the molecule, in constant motion, becomes unstable, like a wheel out of round. It causes the molecule to react with other molecules at the wrong time and place, and tries to "steal" an electron off other molecules to stabilize itself. Radiation sickness is one example of how free radical activity works in the body.

Chlorophyll, the "green blood" of plants, and oxygen producer of our planet through photosynthesis, contains a preform of vitamin A called beta-carotene. This substance is critical to preventing free radical degeneration in the plant. Beta-carotene is also a powerful anti-free-radical agent in the bodies of animals and humans who consume green plants. It is interesting to note that vitamin A in its full form can be toxic in excessive doses, but beta-carotene in its pre-vitamin A form has never been shown to be toxic at any level. That is why grazing animals can consume so much green grass and not develop hypervitaminosis A. But nature did not anticipate current and projected future levels of UV penetration from the sun. The balance has been tipped.

The free radical process occurs as a chain reaction in the molecular structure of the cell when elevated levels of UV stress the plant's ability to protect itself. The unstable free radical molecule collides with another molecule, trying to steal an electron. Like a clumsy drunk spilling a glass, lurching for it, and knocking another over, and then another, the free radical activity causes a frenzy of internal disorder. Trace minerals from mineralized soil, such as zinc, copper, selenium, cobalt, and manganese, as well as beta-carotene and vitamins C and E, are used in plants and humans to form anti-free-radical enzymes. Human enzymes, thought to be formed in the spleen, such as superoxide dismutase and catalase, are examples. They convert free radicals into harmless waste products that are easily eliminated through the liver and kidneys.

Free radicals can be formed in our bodies by a number of physical or chemical insults, or by radiation. UV radiation is a dominant cause of radiation-induced free radicals. Here again, trace minerals and vitamins combine with amino acids to form a protective shield in the form of enzymes.

THE GREENHOUSE EFFECT

The ill-famed "Greenhouse Effect" is an enormous issue emphasizing a global immune system. Here is how it works. The sun's radiant energy reaches the surface of our planet in the form of both visible light and invisible rays including UV light. In the spectrum of energy, these are among the shorter wavelengths. The surface of the planet absorbs these energy waves and gradually releases them as much longer wavelengths called infrared waves. When you feel the warmth radiating off a city street on a summer night or a sandy beach in the evening, those are the infrared waves being released

back into the atmosphere, dissipating into endless space, re-
lieving the planet of this heat.

However, certain gases, including carbon dioxide (CO_2)
and, to a lesser degree, methane (CH_4), trap these waves.
(Methane, though not nearly as plentiful as carbon dioxide,
traps twenty times more heat per ton than carbon dioxide.)
This keeps heat from leaving the Earth's atmosphere, instead
causing it to re-radiate back to the surface of the Earth, much
the same as in a greenhouse.

The Greenhouse Effect is detrimental because it causes
more heat than the Earth can handle to be trapped within its
atmosphere.

Where is all this carbon dioxide that causes the Greenhouse
Effect coming from? The burning of fossil fuels such as coal,
gasoline, and oil creates a huge surplus of carbon dioxide.
Forest fires and volcanic eruptions are other global sources
of immense carbon dioxide release into the atmosphere.
The huge beef cattle feed lots in ranching areas release ex-
cess amounts of methane into the atmosphere from animal
waste.

The massive vegetation on the land and in the oceans
would tend to consume much of the carbon dioxide, the most
abundant greenhouse gas. But the precise ratio of trees-
to-carbon dioxide has been dangerously altered by commercial foresting without replanting. We will discuss these
phenomena in the sections that follow.

Furnaces of Industry and the Greenhouse Effect

Our planet is a carbon-based life form. The perilous, man-
made imbalance between carbon stored in the land and its
massive release, through combustion into the air combining
with oxygen to form carbon dioxide, was first noted in 1896
by Swedish Nobel Prize-winning chemist Svante Arrkenias.
He warned that the furnaces of industry and urban life might
make life on Earth impossible. We all contribute to this un-
sustainable way of life because the furnaces of industry are
simply producing the goods and products that we have de-
manded in the marketplace.

Eight of the top nine corporations listed in *Fortune Magazine*'s Fortune 500 for 1989 are prime producers of the products that directly cause this massive shift in the Earth's climate and the Greenhouse Effect. The top nine in ascending order are: General Motors (automobiles, trucks, and heavy machinery), Ford Motor (automobiles, trucks, and heavy machinery), Exxon (oil, gas, and coal), International Business Machines (non-primary contributor to the Greenhouse Effect), General Electric (electrical generating facilities and equipment), Mobil Oil (gas and oil), Chrysler (automobiles and trucks), Texaco Inc. (oil and gas), and Du Pont (industrial chemicals including ozone-destroying CFCs).

These, the largest American corporations, grew to be as large and powerful as they are by becoming the bedrock upon which our energy-gluttonous civilization stands. They cannot be faulted for responding to the demands of a free marketplace. It is *we*, the consumers of this Greenhouse Effect-creating lifestyle, who have created the suppliers. The consuming public has always rejected the perceived inconveniences associated with alternative clean sources of energy.

Often the public, guided by the mass media exploiting a hot story, singles out highly visible environmental disasters caused by an act of negligence or abuse. But this is a symptomatic view of a systemic problem, and only serves to vent anger at one specific environmental incident.

For example, the ship responsible for the worst oil spill in United States history, the Exxon oil tanker *Valdez*, is now a household name after having spewed ten million gallons of crude oil into Alaska's pristine Prince William Sound in April 1989. As environmentally devastating and tragic to fish and wildlife as this is, it is hardly the most important point. We, the oil-devouring society, ordered the oil and, like a bumbling waiter, Exxon just spilled it. Where is our responsibility in the matter? If Exxon had not "dropped the tray" in filling our order, so to speak, we would have burned the oil and released hundreds of tons of carbon dioxide, carbon monoxide, and other deleterious substances into the atmosphere. No one ever spilled sunlight in creating solar energy.

The Forests and the Greenhouse Effect

The relationship between deforestation and the Greenhouse Effect is an obvious one. But Americans seem to be able to see only distant objects clearly when it comes to environmental causes.

Unfortunately, a vigorous green life, needed to remove carbon dioxide and create oxygen, is vanishing from this planet at a staggering rate. Whether cleared to raise cheap beef in Central or South America, or to make room for our cars at the mall, trees—the great lungs of the earth—are sacrificed. Foresters estimate that every ton of living tree extracts one and a half tons of carbon dioxide from the air, while giving back a ton of oxygen. A single person needs about one pound of oxygen per day. Deciduous trees, with broad leaf area, consume many times more carbon dioxide and give back more oxygen than do the thin needle conifers (pines). Chestnut trees, now rapidly disappearing, have been measured at sixty acres of leaf area. But the trees with the greatest leaf area require the most minerally abundant and moist soils to sustain their massive feeding. Therefore, as erosion, acid rain, fires, lumbering, and development deplete our forests, the thin needle conifers are becoming ubiquitous. The proud maples of New England and eastern Canada are struggling to survive, and one only needs to chart the high price of pure maple syrup to measure the health of the maple forests.

The Rain Forests: Splinter in America's Eye

Many documentaries graphically showing the rain forest annihilation in the Amazon jungle have been aired on network, cable, and public TV. Newspaper and magazine articles regularly appear about Brazil, Costa Rica, Indonesia, and other nations that have cleared or are clearing their rain forests. Predictably, these have created a public outcry, and congressional panels have journeyed to some of these places to plead with the local governments for restraint and restrictions. Talk about exchanging Third World debt for preserving rain forest wilderness has swirled about the media and environmental coalitions. Ask almost any American in 1989 and he will quickly say, "I am an environmentalist." She will say, "We must save the rain forests." This has become a fashionable attitude. But what do the American facts say about our own precious rain forest in the Northwest?

The American rain forest is a sprawling expanse of coastal evergreens that spreads from northern California to southeastern Alaska. These trees comprise the largest and oldest timberlands in the United States. The *New York Times* in 1989 reported, "The last ancient forests are being logged at the rate of 60,000 acres a year—three times the annual harvest at the height of the post-war building boom." The vast majority of the timber is for foreign export (as is Third World rain forest timber). These timberlands are part of The National Forest Trust System, created in 1905 by President Theodore Roosevelt to preserve our heritage and environment. The United States Forest Service has opened up the United States rain forest to logging companies as never before. Perhaps their new logo should picture Smokey Bear with a chain saw. The Wilderness Society fears that in just fifteen years the American rain forests, the rare animal and plant life existing there today, will be gone forever. This is likely to happen.

A valorous witness to the wholesale destruction of the vanishing Western American Wilderness was author Edward Abbey, who died in 1989. Here is his cogent view of modern values at work in our mountains and forests, slashing and paving our link with the Earth:

> The American West has not given us, so far, sufficient men to match our mountains. Or not since the death of Crazy Horse, Sitting Bull, Dull Knife, Red Cloud, Chief Joseph, Little Wolf, Red Shirt, Gall, Geronimo, Chochise, Tenaya (to name but a few), and their comrades. With their defeat died a bold, brave, heroic way of life, one as fine as anything recorded history has to show us. . . .
>
> Instead of mountain men, we are cursed with a plague of diggers, drillers, borers, grubbers; of asphalt-spreaders, dam-builders, overgrazers, clear-cutters, and strip miners, whose object seems to be to make our mountains match our men—making molehills out of mountains for a race of rodents—for the rat race.

Even as America's once-revered forests fall to the chain saw, we criticize very poor nations for their wreckless environmental ways. Fed up with caravans of reporters and news crews, the mayor of one town carved out of the Amazon rain forest repeated in published interviews his advice to the Americans to "reforest Vietnam" if they wanted to cleanse their consciences. He told the *New York Times* that America "burned Vietnam's forests with napalm and other bombs. . . . Now they want to wash their consciences by blocking the development of Brazil." The use of *Agent Orange* as a jungle defoliant in Vietnam was the ultimate in instant deforestation. What the world is saying back to the United States in essence is "Actions speak louder than words."

On March 19, 1989, the United Nations Economic and Social Commission for Asia and the Pacific released a study blaming most of Asia's 1988 "natural disasters" (*How strange to call them "natural"!*) primarily on deforestation. "The phenomena of floods, mudslides, even earth quakes can be directly related to deforestation," the United Nations report stated. I do believe that we are finally doing more than talking about the weather; I believe we are creating it.

In an appeal to my fellow Coloradoans (at least 110 percent of whom claim they are environmentalists!), I submitted the following letter to the editor of the *Denver Post*, which they printed during the 1988 Christmas season.

> Driving along Colorado highways, particularly in the mountains, one witnesses the stream of people in cars and trucks returning from the wilderness with their plunder: dead young pine trees to decorate the homes of Christians for about three weeks.
>
> Concerned Earth watchers are pleading with developing nations around the globe to stop the deadly deforestation that is causing environmental havoc, ranging from massive flooding, soil erosion, desertification, to global oxygen deficiency and the lack of CO_2 absorption, which is the primary Greenhouse Effect gas. How can we ask these countries to find alternative ways to handle their financial problems other than destroying their forests, when hundreds of millions of Christians celebrate their holiest birthday by cutting down young trees and put-

ting them, of all places, in their house. Placing a dead decorated tree in the home, to me, considering the present precarious state of the world's forests, is of questionable taste and is unquestionably environmentally wasteful. It is time to find more suitable symbols to express our beliefs.

The next day at about 9 a.m., talk show host Mike Rosen read the letter on Denver's major talk radio station, News Radio 85-KOA. Coincidentally, I had just tuned in my radio in the middle of it. Both callers and the show's host ridiculed the letter with bitter sarcasm and dismissed it as crazy. "Should we also ban pumpkins on Halloween?" one caller railed. "No," I thought to myself, "but you should eat lots of Halloween candy in hopes that Darwin was right and you will become extinct." While I did receive some personal phone calls of support, the feedback was quite revealing.

It would seem that, even in an environmentally sensitive state like Colorado, the home of the Rocky Mountains, the average citizen is not willing to make personally either symbolic or real modifications in lifestyle (or is it a death-style?) to preserve the environment. Their attitude appears to be, "It's okay to pressure people who speak another language and live thousands of miles away, but don't ask me to change what I do." The sad thing is, America has always stood for leadership. And that means "leading the ship." And that means doing it first.

Climatic Influences of the Greenhouse Effect

So, wrecklessly along we go. While most agree the Greenhouse Effect is real, no one knows for certain its precise outcome. A majority of climatologists claim that it is causing us to enter a serious warming trend that will bring drought, crop failure, growing deserts, disease, and fresh water shortage. But a few respected scientists disagree. Their theory is a rarely publicized deviation in scenario concerning long-term weather consequences. On the theory of warming, this small nucleus of climatologists says, "Not so." In fact, their prediction is quite the opposite.

The Alternative Greenhouse Scenario: The Big Chill

John Hamaker, previously mentioned regarding rock dust, offers a plausible alternative theory to a global warming caused by the Greenhouse Effect. Hamaker thinks the Greenhouse Effect will ultimately, but soon, make the world colder. Much colder. In fact, he believes a new ice age will result, decimating civilized life on our planet. His theory, while far from having been accepted by mainstream science, has been accepted by some prominent climatologists in the United States and Europe.

Hamaker says the results of the Greenhouse Effect are not the same throughout the planet. Different regions react differently. This varied reaction to the Greenhouse Effect creates large temperature differentials between regions, consequently creating massive climatic shifts as laws of thermodynamics come into play. Hamaker states that the greenhouse gases build up primarily in the temperate mid-latitude regions where they are produced, increasingly warming these areas. As the temperature differential between the polar and mid-latitude regions widens, tremendous winds are generated. These high-velocity winds are caused by the rising of the hot air while the freezing air from the poles descends under it. Hot air rises, cold air falls. Hamaker predicts that the turbulence created by these enormous bodies of air flowing rapidly in opposite directions will spawn ever more fierce hurricanes, tornadoes, and severe weather patterns. True to his forecast, Hurricane Gilbert in 1988 was the worst hurricane ever recorded in the Western Hemisphere. If Hamaker is right, this is just a sample of things to come. But how does this trigger an ice age?

Normally, the rising warm air over the tropics would be somewhat cooled by the massive rain forest cover at those latitudes. As these rain forests are cut down, they do not remove carbon dioxide from the air, thus adding to the Greenhouse Effect and a hotter atmosphere. The higher temperatures cause increased evaporation of the tropical oceans. This hotter rising air is therefore increasingly more dense with moisture. As the upper jet streams intensify, moving away from the tropics because of the cold polar air racing in beneath it, they carry this moisture toward the poles. Great clouds form, resulting in tremendous precipitation in the higher latitudes. Ever more flood-causing rain falls in the higher regions of the temperate zones, and dense snow falls at the colder polar zones. The snow pack expands as the equatorial moisture-laden air continues to transfer water from the warm oceans to the ice-capped regions. This process inches forward indefinitely as the polar regions grow, forcing their cold air ever more toward the temperate latitudes. The result: another ice age. Sound incredible?

Geologists agree that ice ages come in cycles approximately every 100,000 years, last for about 90,000 years, and are followed by an interglacial warming period lasting about 10,000 years. *Our present interglacial warm period is estimated to have begun just over 10,000 years ago.* Translated into geological time frames, an ice age is due any minute.

This process, says Hamaker, will create ever-colder temperatures in the temperate, food-growing regions of the planet. The impact on global food supply will be devastating. Right now, world wheat reserves are at a fifteen-year low.

Hamaker believes that an all-out global effort to remineralize the Earth's soils (with rock dust) and the planting of billions of trees, coupled with the elimination of fossil fuel burning, and the development of alternative sources of power (for example, hydrogen, solar, and wind) can restore the carbon balance between the land and atmosphere. This, he believes, if accomplished very soon, would reverse the Greenhouse Effect and could stop the coming ice age.

"An astonishing service for humanity. A complete world view which has been sitting under the noses of many scientists, and which all of them seem to have overlooked." This is the response to Hamaker's work of Kenneth Watt, professor of environmental studies, University of California, and author of the *Annual Review of the Environment* for the *Encyclopaedia Britannica*.

That the United States is in fact, on average, cooling, is finding its way into scientific literature. The March 20, 1989 issue of the *Journal of Geophysical Research* (Volume Number D3) presented a report entitled "Historical Temperature Trends in the United States and the Effect of Urban Population Growth." In compiling data for this report, Arizona State University climatological researchers Robert Balling and Sherwood Idso, along with the United States Water Conservation Laboratory, researched the records of 1,200 weather stations in small towns around the United States. Their findings pointed to a general overall cooling. Why the discrepancy with mainstream science reports? According to these Arizona climatologists, the "Urban Heat Island Effect" has been severely warping weather records used by most researchers. The presence of civilization with its trillions of tons of concrete and massive emissions has created micro-ecosystems that do not accurately reflect what is occurring overall. In a phone conversation, Sherwood Idso told me there is great closed-mindedness in the scientific community to any scenario other than a global warming. Even clear presentation of objective facts, for the most part, falls on deaf ears. Idso also believes that the massive carbon dioxide atmosphere is overstimulating plant growth. This could result in more rapid depletion of available soil nutrition in forests and dense vegetation regions as roots search more furiously for mineral nutrition. His book, *CO_2 and Global Change: Earth in Transition*, explores possibilities.

For a full presentation on the ice age theories of John Hamaker, refer to *The Survival of Civilization* by John Hamaker and Don Weaver; *The End* by Larry Ephron; and a one-hour video called *Stopping the Coming Ice Age*. These can all be obtained from People for a Future, 2000 Center Street, Berkeley, CA 94704. Telephone (415) 524-2700.

Here we are nearing the end of the twentieth century, the century that offered so much promise of hope and human enlightenment, and through our conscious actions, the immune system of the planet and mankind is breaking down. The planet, in integrated essence, is our immune system. We are defenseless without it. We are systematically destroying the machinery of the immune system of the planet and wondering why we have diseases like AIDS and cancer. We are all part of a living whole, so we cannot escape the fact that our immune system is under siege from unfiltered solar radiation, the sun. The poisoned and depleted Mother Earth below and the unfiltered Father Sun above, the parents who nor-

mally fill us with the life force, are going to be the murderers
of their unseeing and uncaring children. It is right to take
this personally, because no matter how widespread the problem, each will personally suffer the consequences.

TAKE RESPONSIBILITY FOR OUR ENVIRONMENT

Malignant melanoma, a skin cancer that spreads like wildfire,
one of the most lethal forms of cancer, is up 80 percent in
recent decades. This is related to man-made interferences
with the immune system of the planet, especially the ozone
layer depletion. Be it unfiltered radiation from the sun above,
or radiation from nuclear disasters like Chernobyl on the
ground, it is the out-of-sync actions of mankind that are
wearing down the planet and humankind.

There are ways to protect ourselves, to a certain extent,
from these kinds of things. I know I have presented a disturb-
ingly negative picture here, but we have to know the facts.
I'm not trying to frighten you; I'm trying to offer some facts
and instruction. The popular media leads us to believe that
the heroes of modern science are in the laboratories right now
looking through microscopes, testing animals, researching,
trying computer programs, nearing solutions. But, like the
Soviet Five Year Plans, or the blatherings of our own misguided politicians, these empty promises are not new.

On a positive note, most of what we need to be perfectly
well, whole, and healthy is already discovered, is already
available on the planet. I see no evidence of some begrudging
God up there, withholding information until the last desperate moment, and, just in the nick of time, sending out a little
gem of lifesaving wisdom. No. The answers are here, known,
teachable, practical, and doable.

Application is what we need. If people applied the teach-
ings of Dr. Bernard Jensen, just think of how it would increase their general wellness and resistance. Don't look to
Dan Rather to tell you about it on the evening news, because
he's usually looking for it from the people who created the
problem. How much televised objectivity is given to alternative approaches to health, energy, and the environment?
There were men like Dr. William Albrecht, men like Dr. Royal

Lee, and other men and women researchers throughout the world, who have already given us the necessary information to achieve and maintain well-being.

MEET THE TOXIC CONTAMINATION HEAD-ON

A question I am frequently asked was put particularly well by a guest in the audience when I spoke at a conference last year. She said, "In Indiana there was a case involving a dump full of discarded batteries. The battery acid contaminated the water and soil in that area and needed cleaning up. My brother, an engineer, worked on this project and he had to help wash the soil. What are we to do with all this poison? Isn't it necessary to develop technology that will enable us to clean up the air, water, and land?"

The answer is, of course, *yes*, but keep in mind that the amount of agricultural toxic pollution is greater than all other forms of pollution added together! Because of the incredible degree of toxic contamination we've caused, such as in this place in Indiana, environmental engineers need to find ways to clean it up. But the greatest mistake of all would be to rely on clean-up techniques that give us a false security to go on living in our polluting ways. What about not producing all this environmental poison? That is more important in the long run than cleaning it up. Consider the statistics in Table 5.1. It reports what is known to be dumped by industry into the Mississippi River annually. The global environmental group Greenpeace provided the information.

This corridor of cancer was once called "the father of all waters" by President Abraham Lincoln, and is the water supply for scores of our most populated cities. Is it a question of clean-up or, more fundamentally, when do we say, "Enough is enough. Not another drop!" If the river could speak, it would just say, "No." Unfortunately, the EPA and the state governments have said, "Apply here for license to pollute."

There is a way for this planet to detoxify, just as there are ways to detoxify the body. Look to the human body to find the engineering and biochemical principles needed in the outer environment. After all, would anyone question the precision and effectiveness of our design?

Table 5.1 Industrial Wastes Dumped
in the Mississippi River
(per year)

Industrial Waste	Quantity (in pounds)
Aluminum	11,473,440
Copper	921,000
Nickel	732,973
Chloroform	104,000
Polynuclear Aromatic Hydrocarbons	62,877
Atrazine	61,693
Dichloromethane	42,801
Alachlor	31,020
Carbon Tetrachloride	10,700
Chromium	10,700
Trichloroethylene	10,700

Source: Greenpeace

What is the first thing you do when you have a highly contaminated substance? You contain it. You insulate it. That's why a cut develops pus. That's why you amass water when you injure your knee and it becomes swollen. The first thing the natural intelligence of the body does is to build a protective barricade, insulating and isolating the contaminated substance so that it does not get into the general stream of things, until that material can be broken down enzymatically, reabsorbed, or eliminated.

Then, of course, we have the liver, which will take these highly contaminated substances, store them, or decontaminate them with enzymes or Kupffer cells and put them in the bile which soon leaves the body. The pollution and contamination needs cleaning up and needs isolating, but that is merely a fraction of the problem. It's a lot easier to contain a waste site. You just say, "No one can be here for a hundred years," or whatever it takes. But how do you contain the state of Kansas? How do you contain the state of Texas? How much poison lies in their soils?

There is only one way. How do you get off drugs? Former first lady Nancy Reagan suggested that you just say, "No!"

You have to quit cold turkey, but you have to do it with understanding. When you pull a crutch away from someone, you'd better have something else there that can support them. If they've been relying on the crutch, there's an atrophying of muscle, and there's a dependency. Something must be replaced. We know what needs replenishment.

There are ways to restore the land that are well known. My land in Colorado was nothing but weeds. It wouldn't even grow grass. But now it is restored. I know farmers down in Louisiana who had so much DDT on their land because of previous cotton farming there, that part of their whole process was not planting food crops for five years. They just planted crops that put nutrients in the soil and then plowed them back in; planted cover crops to protect the soil and plowed them back in. As trace minerals were added, worms returned. They were building new and richer topsoil. It's going to take some years, but it can be done. Nothing's going to happen until there's the will and the understanding. But our backs are against the wall. The first thing to overcome is the mentality of our addiction to chemicals and their poisoned promises.

6

Updating Notions of What Causes Disease

At this point, we should consider our own bodies directly and how we are designed brilliantly to deal with these problems. Do not think that you must be a doctor to understand principles of how your body works. You do not need to be a Swiss watchmaker to know how to tell time. To understand our human body's immune system, we must understand that it is not a single organ or even one system. Rather, as we have noted, it is an alliance of organs and systems, working together to create an overall immune function. Just as the police, fire, and sanitation departments are independent systems within a larger city government, they coordinate and communicate to create an overall function that is for the protection of the whole. The T-lymphocytes, and the thymus gland that creates them, are the more famous and front-line parts of the immune system. But there are still postwar medical textbooks that say the thymus gland is a useless atrophied endocrine gland after childhood. Naturalist doctors have long supported the idea that the thymus gland must always be nourished with the right nutrients and herbs because it functions throughout our lifetime. If the thymus gland was not continuously active in creating immunity, why was it the foremost obstacle to be overcome in the procedure of organ transplants? It is the thymus that sets up the rejection of the foreign implanted organs because "they do not belong to this body."

Researchers are exploring nonsensical methods such as freezing our youthful, thymus-derived T-lymphocytes and re-injecting them back into our older bodies. The November 1988 issue of *Longevity* magazine quotes one immune system researcher, who said, "I feel strongly that if we could counteract the shrinkage of the thymus, we would not only sustain the activity of the immune system but might extend the life span as well." Here is another example of highly funded medical researchers overlooking prior nutritional research hoping to find exotic (translation: "expensive") chemical substitutes.

Thirteen years earlier, in the September 1975 issue of the journal *Infectious Diseases*, Dr. Eli Seifter, professor of biochemistry of the New York-based Albert Einstein College of Medicine, wrote, "When the body is subjected to stress, the immune response suffers and the thymus gland, which is vital to the cell's protection, tends to shrink. *Vitamin A increases the size of the thymus which apparently stimulates the body's defense against disease* [emphasis added]."

The thymus's shrinking comes *after* disease and malnutrition. As medical researchers return to the "useless gland" (as it is called in many post-World War II texts) for answers, nutrition will be the answer. The respected Weizmann Institute in Tel Aviv, Israel, reported as far back as 1976 the successful use of animal thymus gland extracts to treat infectious diseases in children not responding to antibiotics. Dr. Royal Lee reported similar findings twenty years before that.

Yes, the immune system has some key players, but it functions across a broad range of the body's systems. When we have an infection of some kind, it is because there is a high count of pathogenic bacteria or viruses concentrated somewhere in the body, trying to break down dead or diseased tissue. I am not saying that the germ theory of medicine is totally without basis but, rather, without perspective.

The germ theory of medicine is a nineteenth-century concept, promoted by Louis Pasteur before vitamins, trace elements, and other nutrients had even been discovered. The germ theory is still believed to be the central cause of disease, because around it exists a colossal supportive infrastructure of commercial interests that built multi-billion-dollar industries based upon this theory. To the scientific satisfaction of many in the health field, it has long been disproven as the primary cause of disease. Germs are, rather, an effect of disease.

Nevertheless, like dogs chasing their own tails, scientists go cross-eyed looking in microscopes (or should I say "microbescopes") to discover new disease-causing germs. In January 1989, the Atlanta Center for Disease Control reported that at least 200 different viruses can cause the common cold. A little common sense about the common cold would reveal the nonsense of that assertion. In my opinion, that statement does more to beg forgiveness from the chemical approach to disease than to show enlightened understanding about cause and effect. Surely, the guy on the street with a cold cannot fault medicine for not having a drug to cure his cold when he would need 200 different chemicals aimed at interfering with all the possibilities of the so-called "cause" of his problem. One ponders geometrically for a moment; if 200 viruses can cause the simple common cold, think how many more evil microbes they believe must cause cancer.

Yet, false hope springs eternal in the human mind. In March 1989, medical researchers announced that they were perhaps five to ten years away from a cold-preventing drug. This hope derived from a discovery of the place in the cell attacked by the *rhino* virus, which they blame for one-third of all colds. This presumes, of course, that viruses actually attack cells rather then just act as a scavenger cleaning up the waste, which we will shortly discuss. If, hypothetically, they could produce a cold-inhibiting drug, just what would the side effects be of stopping the elimination of all the cell waste thrown off by cold symptoms? If you stop a cold, you stop what the body is accomplishing by the action of a cold.

Is it not ironic, indeed pathetic, that as human beings, the potentially highest form of life expression on this planet, we have built the vast pharmaceutical industry for the central purpose of poisoning the lowest form of life on the plant— germs? As Dr. Royal Lee said almost thirty years ago, "One of the biggest tragedies of human civilization is the precedence of chemical therapy over nutrition. It's a substitution of artificial therapy over natural, of poisons over food, in which we are feeding people poisons [drugs], trying to correct the reactions of starvation."

Harmful germs are a natural reaction to starved tissue. Nowadays, the medical obsession with killing microbes would stun even the "father of antibiotics," Nobel-Prize-laureate Selman Waksman, M.D., who wrote in 1954, "It is usually not recognized that for every injurious or parasitic microbe there are dozens of beneficial ones. Without the latter, there would be no bread to eat nor wine to drink, no fertile soils and no potable waters, no clothing and no sanitation. One can visualize no form of higher life without the existence of the microbes. They are the universal scavengers. They keep in constant circulation the chemical elements which are so essential to the continuation of plant and animal life."

So germs or microbes flourish as savengers at the site of disease. Enlightened understanding is that they are not the cause of the disease, any more than flies and maggots cause garbage. Flies, maggots, and rats do not cause garbage but rather feed on it, and that's why I refer to the germ theory of medicine as "the rat theory of garbage." That is, if germs cause disease, then rats must cause garbage. Show me a town that's full of rats and I'll show you a town that's full of garbage. I'll show you a town with a sanitation problem, I guarantee it. Take me to your cockroaches. Come to think of it, I always see firemen at burning buildings. . . .

ARE WE MISSING THE POINT?

Think of this for a moment. The immune system of the human body is remarkably sophisticated. It makes the most advanced computer software in the world look like a child's toy.

The immune system of plants is comparatively simple, isn't it? Once you understand it, it's not that difficult to explain.

What happens when we take an antibiotic (penicillin or its derivatives) into our bodies? Penicillin is a specific antibacterial secretion of a fungus. Penicillin was seen as a great miracle and, certainly, when introduced in the middle of World War II, many soldiers' lives were saved because of penicillin. However, there's always a price to pay down the road when you do something left-handed with nature. When we use a plant's method of killing bacteria in our own bodies, *we reduce our human level of immune function to that of a vegetable.*

ANTIBIOTICS AND THE LOSS OF IMMUNITY

Antibiotics in our bodies cannot tell the cops from the robbers. With no discretion, they kill friendly as well as harmful bacteria. The vast majority of bacteria are helpful, actually working for us, like the microflora in our intestines. Destruction of this microflora produces a common side effect of antibiotic therapy in humans and animals: diarrhea. Overgrowth of the yeast organism, *Candida albicans*, is another common side effect of antibiotic therapy. Our own immune systems, now placed on welfare by the medical doctor, decide not to work. A false sense of temporary resistance is acquired by the body. The antibiotic can also weaken our immune system by creating certain B-vitamin deficiencies. The micro-intestinal flora, the friendly bacteria that protect the GI tract, synthesize certain B vitamins such as B_{12}, the anti-pernicious-anemia vitamin (made from the trace mineral organic cobalt). Minute levels of this powerful vitamin, measured in micrograms (thousandths of a gram), maintain the health of billions of red blood cells that sustain our life. Antibiotics kill the friendly bacteria that manufacture vitamin B_{12} in the gut. Where is the logic behind depressing our immune system to fight an infection artificially—especially when we run the increased risk of developing super strains of pathogenic bacteria that have mutated to circumvent the antibiotic? These super strains are showing up in more and more hospitals, known as "super infections."

An antibiotic is a plant's immune system. Why do we use another species' method of protecting ourselves? We have our own, more-sophisticated internal mechanism for self-defense. Animals and humans do not produce antibiotics, nor do they need to, if their endocrine, immune, and nervous systems have the mineral, vitamin, protein, and enzyme substances found in foods grown on mineral-rich soil. Armed with these tools, the Earth's highest forms of life—humans and animals—are well equipped to fight the Earth's lowest forms of life—bacteria and virus. Let's learn how that works, strengthen it, and use it effectively. It has kept human beings surviving for thousands of centuries. Nature's track record for being right should inspire our trust.

WHY WE HEAR SO MUCH ABOUT
CANDIDA ALBICANS

I want to stress here the cause of one of the most common conditions we see today. So many people have suddenly realized that their body has been overcome by a yeast organism overpopulating the gut, *Candida albicans*. I don't have to spend much time with it because, in a sense, I've previously explained the principles of its occurrence.

We normally have yeast in our body. Yeast is a type of fungi. We're exposed to yeast all the time. I never met a yeast I wouldn't eat. Yeasts are fine, healthy, ecologically safe, and balanced substances. The problem arises when any substance in the body gets out of balance; then it becomes harmful. An overgrowth of *Candida albicans* in the digestive tract is reported to create severe allergy symptoms: headaches, skin eruptions, chronic fatigue, digestive distress, and general immune-system frailty.

We are foolishly using antibiotics in the livestock food chain. Where is the antibiotic-laden livestock destined? It finds its way into the mouths of human beings. Do you know who the largest purchasers of antibiotics are? Livestock food makers such as Purina Corporation are the world's largest because they put it in much of their animal feed: poultry feed, rabbit feed, cattle feed, as well as others. Antibiotics are in all pork; pigs are fed more antibiotics than any other animals.

Why? Because pigs are dirty; they get a lot of bacteria. Then, of course, there is the medical profession's generally acknowledged excessive and obsessive use of antibiotics. This all represents a man-made frontal assault on the human immune system. Plus, it gives pathogenic bacteria an opportunity to mutate into even more deadly, resistant forms. As stated previously, this matter of bacterial mutation has been already seen as "super infections" in hospitals where the overuse of antibiotics is often the norm.

This sheds more light on what I referred to earlier. When you take an antibiotic for infection, you may get over that strep throat quickly, or you may not. Should you be lucky— just don't count on it—should that even occur, you'll pay a dear price later. That big bill comes because you have knocked out the body's bacterial line of defense, the intestinal flora.

An overgrowth of *Candida albicans* occurs because *Candida* is an opportunistic yeast organism. Only when kept in check by competing microorganisms will this yeast stay in a balanced population. The Atlanta Center for Disease Control lists Candidiasis as an official symptom of AIDS. Why is that? Because the AIDS victim has so little immune function that the *Candida* does not have anything controlling it. With nothing competing with or protecting against it in the gut (or vaginal tract, where it is a common cause of yeast infections, a common side effect of antibiotics), it begins to flourish, and it expands higher up in the GI tract. The primary question is not how to kill this invader, but where were the protective factors? The protectors, *acidophilus bacilli*, *bifidus*, and *acidophilus* yeast, were probably destroyed by antibiotics, chlorinated water, and constant consumption of junk foods. A diet high in sugar would also spur further yeast growth because it is such a simple carbohydrate food that the yeast can thrive on it.

There are any number of good books you can find in health food stores describing dietary outlines for *Candidiasis*. As with most dietary approaches to health, there are differences of opinion. Ultimately, you alone should learn how to take responsibility for diet and lifestyle. Your digestion is at a different level from someone else's. One person, for instance, may not be able to have any fruit for a while; someone else might be able to have some. Learning to take control and discern what it is that can bring your body back into balance is part of the healing process. You know the principles, and the principles haven't changed, but the application has to fit your individuality.

CORRECTING THE *CANDIDA* IMBALANCE

It's good to take *acidophilus* if you have excessive *Candida* in the gut because it helps to restore a natural balance, but it will not kill *Candida*, because bacteria are not strong enough. The need is to create an environment so clean that the *Candida* starve while putting stronger healthy flora in. That's the best approach. Under a doctor's care, in extreme cases, there is the option to take a prescription drug such as nystatin, which will go in there and kill it indiscriminately by sterilizing the gut. I'm not recommending you do this, except in the worst situations, and then only if you fortify later with healthy bacteria and enzymes to repopulate and keep clean the GI tract.

The first thing you should do with candidiasis is get your digestive tract back in order. This is foremost. You want to get a clean digestive tract. One step toward that is to completely digest your food. You need to have plenty of digestive enzymes and hydrochloric acid (HCl) in the stomach. As I mentioned, most people with digestive problems don't have too much HCl in their stomach, they have too little, regardless of what all the antacid commercials say. Without HCl, food begins to ferment in the stomach.

The stomach is simply a hydrochloric-acid machine, and, therefore, because of the protection it renders, is actually a part of the immune system. Do you know what the stomach keeps you immune from? Parasites. The eggs of parasitic worms, or insects, or harmful bacteria, may be inadvertently swallowed. One might pet a dog or a cat and pick up some parasite eggs, invisible to the eye, on the finger. Then upon putting your finger in your mouth for some reason, you may swallow the eggs. When I lived in Louisiana, we used to go out and pick strawberries early in the morning—endless strawberry patches. We'd put ten in the bag and one in the mouth. Many times I was amazed at how big half a worm could look in a strawberry. "Man, he must have been huge. Look how big half of him is," I'd think to myself. Then I'd realize where the other half was. Fortunately, I had plenty of HCl in my stomach to destroy any parasites.

Let's use the analogy of the Garden of Eden. What guards the Garden of Eden? The sword of fire that swings every which way. If the body is the temple of the living God, what guards our Garden of Eden? The stomach, the acid machine. The organ of fire. It has one function in life, to make HCl. The only biological reason the stomach lives is to make HCl! Do we want to take that one function away from it? There are pharmaceutical companies making billions just in their efforts to destroy the function of the human stomach.

WHAT CAUSES HEARTBURN

When the stomach digests, it churns. The more HCl it has, the less it has to churn, because the churning action is just a means of mixing the HCl, juices, pepcinogen, and enzymes in contact with the food. If there's no HCl, the food begins to rot. It begins to break down through the process of fermentation. After all, it's 98.6°F, dark, and wet in there. Anything would rot in that environment without enzymatic and digestive juices preventing the decay.

There's a little HCl left in the stomach, so the stomach starts to churn harder and harder to put the juices in contact with the decaying food matter. At some point in this deficient digestive process, a fermentation process starts, and organic acids of fermentation develop. These are deviant acids; they do not belong in the human body. They are by-products of fermentation. They're very stinging. As the stomach starts to churn harder and harder, some of it regurgitates back up into the esophagus, and the organic acids of fermentation, along with whatever small amount of HCl remains, sting that epithelial lining. This process is what produces the symptoms of heartburn.

What caused the heartburn? HCl deficiency. You then take an antacid, if you're so inclined, and the antacid immediately cools you down because it neutralizes any acid, including the deviant organic acids of fermentation. But by doing so you have neutralized what precious little HCl was in the stomach, inhibiting digestion. HCl has been an innocent victim of billions of advertising dollars aimed at blaming it to sell antacids.

Next, this undigested food mass enters the duodenum (gut). It leaves through the pyloric valve about three hours after it has entered the stomach, unless it was fruit, which, if eaten alone, takes only about twenty minutes to leave. The food that did not digest in the stomach stays undigested in the gut. Now your liver and your pancreas have to do all your "chewing" (digesting) for you.

HOW UNDIGESTED FOOD BUILDS TOXICITY

This is how the body begins to get toxic, helped along by residues from pesticides and artificial ingredients. Remember, the gut is outside the body. The body only wants the nutrients, it doesn't want the ingested mass. The role of the GI tract is essentially to "separate the wheat from the chaff." Inside the gut, the mass is supposed to be broken down into vitamins, minerals, trace elements, fatty acids, amino acids, and enzymes. You can't make an egg without cracking that shell; the body has to split open the food molecules, break them down, so it can get the gems. The rest is eliminated through the peristaltic action of the bowel. When that does not occur, the GI tract is full of undigested matter. This undigested food mass begins to decay in the thirty feet of GI tract. The decay becomes a host for undesirable pathogenic bacteria scavenging among the waste, some of which will be eventually killed by the yeast, *Candida albicans*, in competition for food. Going back for a moment to the rootlet of the plant where the mycorrhiza live, the bacteria cannot assault the plant because the fungus protects the plant. Fungus will kill bacteria. This is one of the reasons *acidophilus bacilli* is not effective alone when people use it to remedy candidiasis.

NATURE'S SANITATION TEAM

Like HCl, bacteria and viruses, which are cell scavengers, are not there for lack of something better to do. They're there because there is malnourished, enzyme-depleted, diseased, and necrotic tissue. Functioning as nature's biological sanitation department, they must break down and eliminate the sick tissue to prevent further poisoning of the body. If you stop their action, you allow the body's continuous poisoning by the decaying tissue. In other words, if you have a concentration of bacteria living in some organ in the body, you have a staph infection or strep in the throat, for instance, they're there because of unhealthy devitalized tissue and unprocessed metabolic waste. This is linked to the endocrine system, digestive system, and immune system.

Throughout time, an unenlightened mankind assumed that disease was the presence of something evil: ghosts, demons, Satan, curses, spells, the stars, and now, germs. With the enlightened age of unbiased science, the twentieth-century discovery of the vitamins, minerals, trace elements, amino acids, and fatty acids, freed us to realize that disease is not the presence of something evil, but rather the lack of the presence of something essential.

SOME SERIOUS NUMBERS

When we pause to look at the numbers, it is clear that modern disease is unimpressed with scientific advancement based upon pharmaceutical approaches. Consider cancer, upon which nothing has been spared in "the war" to research pharmacological, radiological, and surgical treatment. By comparison, almost nothing was spent on natural nutritional therapy. This, despite the United States Surgeon General's July 1988 report, which stated that perhaps two-thirds of all deaths in America in 1987 were related to diet. Also, in 1987, there were more than 900,000 *new* cases of cancer diagnosed. The bottom line of these numbers reveals that you cannot fight disease when you are not causing health.

Between 1965 and 1986, the percentage of adult cigarette smokers dropped 35 percent, from 40 percent to 26.5 percent, and the cancer death rate still kept climbing (see Table 6.1). This is more than slightly interesting because smoking is blamed by medicine as the major cause of cancer.

Table 6.1 United States Deaths From Cancer 1937–1987		

Year	Number of Deaths	Number per 100,000	Percent Increase Over 1937
1937	144,774	112	0
1960	330,700	149	228
1987	476,700	200	303

Source: United States Bureau of Census

We should pause to ponder some relationships in disease etiology. I would not question the strong case linking lung cancer to smoking, yet related factors exist. Before 1930, before the age of toxic agri-chemicals, depleted soils, and junk foods, there was an abundance of long-term heavy smokers, and lung cancer was a very rare disease. Why was lung cancer so rare in the 1920s with a higher percentage of adult male smokers than today? A theory can be made that tobacco growers had long before depleted and exploited their soils. By artificially fertilizing, they grew deficient tobacco plants that attracted all manner of pests and plant disease. Ever-increasing and under-regulated amounts of the highly toxic insecticides like DDT, chlordane, toxaphene, and lindane, and the dangerous organophosphorus compounds were sprayed on tobacco fields. The act of smoking vaporizes these residues as they are inhaled into the smoker's lungs. Add to this a new generation of humans exposed to severe air pollution of lead, chlorinated napthalene, and other waste products of combustion; industry poisons; increased radiation; junk food; and general deficiency; and smoking may just be the proverbial straw that broke the camel's back. In other words, smoking may just be the longest nail in the coffin lid, but not enough to hold it down alone. The first sharp rise in the incidence of lung cancer occurred about 1947. *Enter the postwar twins: the Atomic Age and the Chemical Age.*

The cancer rate has continued to climb despite a 17 percent reduction in alcohol consumption since the 1970s. In 1970, Americans spent $8 billion on legal drugs. In 1986 they spent $31 billion. Are they healthier? The total disease care bill for Americans in 1970 was $75 billion, $349 per person, and 7.4

percent of the gross national product (GNP). In 1986, that number grew to a staggering $458 billion, $1,837 per person, and 11 percent of the GNP. Estimates for 1988 are $511 billion. Medical research, based on the germ theory, rose from $2 billion in 1970 to $8.2 billion in 1986. If we needed more medical doctors, American's sure got them. When John F. Kennedy became president in 1960, our nation had 275,000 M.D.s. By 1985, their ranks had swollen to 577,000. Heart disease is still the Number One killer, and half of all men die of it. While the use of antibiotics increased at a mind-boggling rate, the death rate attributed to septicemia (the presence of bacterial toxins in the blood) has soared. Since 1960, the United States death rate from septicemia jumped from 1.1 person per 100,000 population to 7.2 persons per 100,000 population in 1985, an increased death rate of 555 percent in twenty-five years! The deaths from pneumonia between 1980 and 1985 rose 12 percent. These numbers are from the *Statistical Abstracts of the United States, 1988*, published by the United States Department of Commerce, Bureau of the Census. More money, more doctors, more research, more drugs, more surgery, more disease, more death. Some ask what America has gained by spending these thousands of billions of dollars. I ask, "What have we lost?" The use of poisons to "make war" on disease is somewhat like a firing squad forming a circle with the prisoner in the center.

According to *The Yale-New Haven Hospital Study*, 1.5 million Americans are hospitalized each year with medication reactions, resulting in 100,000 deaths annually. This is buried in the statistics file under "iatrogenic deaths," i.e., "doctor-caused death." That number does not include the almost one thousand deaths that occur each week from what a blue-ribbon medical panel termed "unnecessary operations." That one thousand per week does not include those who die from "necessary operations" such as the six to eight thousand who die annually from complications during gall bladder surgery, called a "routine operation."

"Early detection" has been a major focus in the war on cancer, and billions have been spent on the bad-news-sooner approach. But what good is bad-news-sooner if you still approach the problem from the effect side of cause and effect?

The October 1988 *British Medical Journal* reports a large-scale study (more than 40,000 women during a ten-year period) by Swedish physicians reporting that the use of mammograms, a much-promoted breast cancer early-warning screening technique, may not cause a reduction in breast cancer deaths. It is estimated that 42,000 American women will die of this disease in 1989.

A drug-oriented farming/food system, a drug-oriented medical system, and a society that claims to be fighting a war on drugs (called "our national blight") by arresting teenagers and telling them to "say no" to drugs. That amounts to telling our children to behave in contradiction to every example being set before them on the farm and in the city.

A FAMILIAR EXAMPLE: THE FLU

The word "flu" comes from the Italian word "influenza." In the Middle Ages, people believed that when you had a flu you were under the "influence of the stars." Our modern concept isn't superior. The flu usually hits people when? What time of year? If you notice, most flu epidemics begin when seasons change. Flu gets into full flight when the new season has fully arrived.

If you want to observe a big flu epidemic, just look for some real back-and-forth type of weather, like Indian summers. Let's say October blows cold and snowy as it can here in Colorado. You might get a big snowstorm in October, then in November you can be out in a short-sleeved shirt, hiking. Later in November you get the blizzards again, then December might warm up. Colorado does several hesitation dance steps coming into winter—very mild and then cold and then mild and then cold. That's all you need for the makings of a good flu season. Why? Well, for one thing, because of the thyroid gland. The thyroid is the endocrine gland of metabolism; it helps the body adapt between hot and cold. When the summer is here and it's hot, the thyroid is running comparatively low. We don't need to internally warm the body when it's already externally warm. When it's 80°F or 90°F out, the thyroid can have a long summer rest.

When winter comes along and we need to warm up the engine, so to speak, and get metabolism up, the thyroid releases thyroxin and its other gland-stimulating hormones to speed up metabolism. Many naturalist doctors feel that what occurs at this point, because most people have such unresponsive thyroid glands, is that their bodies do not respond appropriately to such temperature changes. This results in unprocessed metabolic waste, in tissues and from undigested food, accumulating in the system. As waste empties from tissues, it becomes a circulating fluid called "lymph."

This waste builds up in the intestines, liver, kidneys, spleen, and lymph glands, and generally in the blood and tissues. When waste-loaded lymph backs up, it may back up into the spleen, tonsils, and lymph nodes and vessels. The bowels get very sluggish. The body wants to generate heat but the thyroid's not doing it, so we spend two hundred dollars on a down jacket and say, "I'm healthy. I'm warm. The cold doesn't bother me." So, L.L. Bean sells us a warm down jacket, while the unprocessed metabolic waste continues to build up and up. What we get next is the flu.

What does the flu do? It's a turbulent detoxification reaction of the body. Every symptom of a cold or the flu—*every symptom* (the body is not general, it's specific)—every symptom of a cold or the flu is a symptom of detoxification. What are the major symptoms of the flu? High fevers (burning of waste, and bacteria); the pores of the skin open for profuse sweating; diarrhea, the bowels dump; chills, which generate internal heat; vomiting, and coughing up and expectoration of respiratory mucus—all the cleansing actions.

This is a way that the body can violently and quickly get rid of the unprocessed metabolic waste. The waste is a smorgasbord for bacteria. Then we start taking all kinds of antihistamine cold pills and drugs to try to stop the body's correct response because we misunderstand what's going on. Advertising strives to convince us that symptoms are universally bad. In this way, they can sell "relief."

Let's say there's a concentration of strep bacteria in some organ. The T-lymphocytes are in the bloodstream and attack the strep. They go to the infection and stimulate reactions to isolate, cluster, and then destroy this infectious bacteria. They create a free radical molecular instability in the infectious bacteria and cause them to break down. The dead bacteria is transported in lymph and blood for removal. These are methods that the body uses to get dead bacteria out. But the bacteria is just living on the unprocessed metabolic waste and diseased, malnourished, nonresistant tissue in the first place. The immune system can't do anything about the malnourished tissue.

All the immune system is trying to do is get rid of the bacteria that is building up too high. It doesn't mind if there are some bacteria working on waste; it's a matter of degree. The presence of the germs does not constitute the presence of a disease. *Tubercle bacilli* (associated with tuberculosis), for instance, can be cultured in a large percentage of the population that does not have and never will develop tuberculosis. The Centers for Disease Control recently reported that 50 percent of America's homeless population tested positive for tuberculosis, but only 5 percent had any active stage of the disease. When the body is too toxic and weak, there is too much pollution in the system. If the thyroid is unable to stimulate enough metabolic function to help cleanse the tissues, then the bacteria levels build up even higher and the militant lymphocytes or phagocytes go into action. But, these "swat teams" of the immune system require nutrients such as vitamins to be effective. The role of vitamins and minerals in fortifying the body against infection is not generally embraced by pharmaceutical-based medicine. But that has not prevented hundreds of prominent research biochemists from reporting their myriad findings over the last fifty years about infection-fighting aspects of various vitamins.

INFECTION-FIGHTING VITAMINS

The first vitamin ever discovered, vitamin A, was also the first vitamin reported to possess, among other attributes, an anti-infective capability. The authoritative textbook *The Vitamins in Medicine*, Third Edition, by Bicknell and Prescott, reports, "Lowered local resistance to infection is the most important result from the changes in the epithelia brought about by lack of vitamin A."

Bicknell and Prescott say this about vitamin D: "During the last century in England cod-liver oil was greatly prized for its value in tuberculosis which has been amply confirmed, at least as regards vitamin D in the treatment of some forms of tuberculosis, in recent years. This, added to the commonness of catarrhal infections in rickets, and the clinical value of sunshine and ultra-violet light in improving the general condition of consumptive and convalescent patients, has led to a widely held belief that vitamin D increases the bodies resistance to infections."

But, by far, the most heralded vitamin believed to assist in fighting or preventing infection is vitamin C. However, vitamin C, like all the vitamins to varying degrees, has been surrounded by controversy since it was identified in the 1930s. Part of the controversy lay in the fundamental question, "What is a vitamin?" As far as medical science is concerned, vitamin C is nothing more than a chemical called ascorbic acid. But as long ago as the 1940s, Dr. Royal Lee reported evidence that the anti-infection vitamin C *complex* is not just ascorbic acid, but rather that ascorbic acid is the protective preservative "wrapper" or "shell" of the vitamin C *complex*.

Vitamin C was officially discovered in 1937 by the late Dr. Albert Szent Giorgi, in America. Dr. Giorgi, who received the Nobel Prize for his vitamin C work, stated that with just isolated *ascorbic acid*, he had not found the *active* anti-scurvy factor of the C complex. Interesting observation, since "ascorbic" means "anti-scurvy." (In Latin, *a* means "anti," and *scorbutic* means "scurvy".) Ascorbic acid therefore is incorrectly named, but then I guess hammers don't make ham.

For one thing, alone it didn't cure scurvy, which Dr. Giorgi found rather strange, particularly since he'd won the Nobel Prize for it. With isolated ascorbic acid (isolated from Hungarian red pepper), Dr. Giorgi reported, he could not stop the capillary hemorrhaging, so characteristic of scurvy, that he could reliably influence with the "impure" batch of vitamin C-rich food from which the ascorbic acid had been isolated. That's why he went back to the laboratory and discovered vitamin P, the rutin factor of the C complex, which, by the way, exists more in buckwheat (grain and leaf) than it does in citrus fruit. Dr. Royal Lee used the term "synergist" to describe the functional interdependence of biologically related nutrient factors. He described a vitamin as being "biological wheels within wheels"; it never functioned as a vitamin in a chemically isolated form. In this sense, the rutin factor would be a synergist of the ascorbic acid and the vitamin C complex.

Dr. Lee explained that the synergists of a whole C complex included the P factors for capillary and blood vessel wall strength, the J factors, which increased the oxygen-carrying capacity of the blood, and an enzyme at the middle of the C complex called *tyrosinase*. Tyrosinase is an organic copper enzyme and, like all the factors of the C complex, it is protected by the antioxidant, ascorbic acid. Using just the preserving ascorbic acid without the rest of the C complex is like breaking into a bank, stealing the security guard, and leaving the money behind.

Ascorbic acid does not effectively cure or prevent scurvy without its synergists. This is what Dr. Giorgi found out. Interestingly, the nickname of the British people, "Limey's," originates from their sailors' practice of eating limes, currants, and other fresh fruit as well as raw potatoes—all high in the vitamin C complex—to prevent scurvy. However, when the ascorbic acid portion of the Vitamin C complex is found within nature, it functions as an antioxidant preserving the C complex, preventing oxidation. By analogy, I recently heard a lecturer complain that his country of Nepal does not want tourists, but his country does need tourists' money. The tourists transport the money. As a result, he said, there are three main religions in Nepal now: Hinduism, Buddhism, and Tourism. The tourist is the protective carrier of the money; he comes into the country and drops off the money. That's how a preservative antioxidant carries, protects, and drops off the actual vitamin nutrient into the body. But from a commercial standpoint, the idea of "synergists" is not so desirable. By reducing a vitamin complex to a single chemical, chemists can claim to duplicate it in a laboratory and easily mass produce it and sell it as an additive to food or a pill. This would not be possible if they were charged with keeping all the synergistic components intact. As such, vitamins are given single chemical names and single chemical structures for the purpose of selling synthetic vitamins. When you have found the shed skin of a snake, you have not found a snake.

This issue remains a thorn in the side of the synthetic vitamin producer. Lending credence to the "vitamin complex" theory is current research of C. Regnault Roger, chairman of biochemistry at the Conservatoire National des Arts et Métiers in Paris. Writing in the prestigious Swiss science journal *Experientia* in September 1988, Roger calls for a flavonoid classification of Vitamin C_2, a second anti-scurvy factor which is sometimes referred to as vitamin P. He reports that synthetic ascorbic acid fails as a reliable anti-scurvy agent because it does not contain the synergistic flavonoids found with ascorbic acid in foods.

C COMPLEX IS LYMPHOCYTE ARMOR

The body doesn't want ascorbic acid *per se*; it wants the C complex being preserved by ascorbic acid. In 1940, Dr. Lee said that the vitamin C complex is the armor of the lymphocytes. A lymphocyte unarmed with the C complex will fail in its function, it will be impotent, it won't be able to attack and destroy infectious organisms. In laboratories, they're currently taking T-lymphocytes out of the body, trying to supercharge them in test tubes, and then put them back into the body. That's wonderful, isn't it? No, it isn't. It's rather a boring waste of research money and an insult to nature.

Lymphocytic potency appears to be related to copper, the trace mineral at the core of the tyrosinase enzyme. What happens with tyrosinase is very interesting. Dr. Lee taught that if you want to know the most active factor of the C complex, it is organic copper, functioning as the tyrosinase enzyme. There is a medical research report on AIDS stating researchers have found a strange relationship between copper deficiency and ineffective lymphocytes.

When they found lymphocytes that would not kill a pathogenic organism in AIDS victims, it was discovered that they had no copper in them. Perhaps it wasn't the copper, uncombined, that was lacking. What was lacking was the entire C complex, which contains copper, and is normally found on the lymphocyte. Researchers would not find vitamin C complex on that lymphocyte, because all they would recognize as being vitamin C would be ascorbic acid. Once in the body, however, the body sheds the ascorbic acid, the preservative wrapper, the way you shed the peel of an orange; takes the rest of the C complex and places it as the lance of the lymphocyte; and kills bacteria and viruses with it.

Ascorbic acid hasn't anything to do with it except that it's a natural protective factor of the C complex. Researchers are just now finding that without copper there will be no effective lymphocytic activity. Dr. Lee would be very glad to know about this latest finding. Unfortunately, he would have had to wait until 1987 to see what he had already stated in the 1940s proved again by the latest research. There are too many instances like that. That's what I mean when I say let's not wait for the new research to prove what we already know.

In 1939, the same year that Dr. Price published *Nutrition and Physical Degeneration,* the USDA released a report summarizing some startling revelations on nutritional research to date. The government data on vitamin C was pointing to an unambiguous link between vitamin C and the front line of infection resistance in the blood. Dr. Lee's assertions about vitamin C appear well-founded according to this United States Government treatise. In the USDA publication "Food and Life," pages 238–239, the following refers specifically to vitamin C: "At first it was thought that the vitamin was destroyed by the organisms producing the infection, but there is now some evidence that it *actually plays a part in combating the infection because it is necessary for the proper functioning of the blood-serum complement* [T-lymphocyte] [emphasis added]— a substance in the bloodstream that acts as the first line of defense against invasion by harmful agents. It has recently been shown in guinea pigs that the blood-serum complement loses its normal activity in the absence of vitamin C. In human beings too, blood analyses have shown that a high content of vitamin C is accompanied by a high content of blood-serum complement, and vice versa." The USDA report also pointed out that long-term subclinical deficiency of vitamin C would fail to produce the overt recognizable symptoms of scurvy possibly leading to an infectious condition harder to treat: "What may be more serious, the blood system may be weakened to the point where it can no longer resist or fight infections not so easily cured as scurvy."

This USDA report in 1939 would seem to trumpet in an epoch of unparalleled opportunities and insights into the biochemical nature of health and, that bane of human existence, infectious disease. But the very next year, 1940, Howard Florey developed the first practical application of the new "wonder drug," penicillin, and the age of antibiotics was upon us. One may ponder whether the "wonder" was a reference to the colossal sums of money earned by producers of antibiotics.

ASCORBIC ACID—VITAMIN OR pH FACTOR?

Why are there periodic reports of plain ascorbic acid helping to fight various colds and infections? The answer probably lies more in ascorbic acid's pH balance influence (acid/alkaline balance) than any other factor. True to its namesake, ascorbic acid lowers the pH to the acid side of the pH scale. Most infectious pathogenic bacteria thrive in an alkaline pH. This phenomenon of acid/alkaline/bacteria connection was the major subject of investigation about proven folk remedies by a Vermont medical doctor. His curiosity was spurred by a local custom of healthy, hardworking farm families, which was to consume on a regular basis a beverage that was very acidic: a mixture of water and apple cider vinegar with a drop of honey.

In his informative little book, *Folk Medicine*, D. C. Jarvis, M.D., reports about the largely misunderstood pertinence of the acid/alkaline balance to overall resistance to disease. He developed this work by having an associate physician study and prepare a report identifying the pH most favorable to the growth of pathogenic organisms.

Dr. Jarvis and his associate, who worked at a medical school's department of bacteriology, prepared a list entitled "Most Favorable Reaction of Media for Growing Pathogenic Bacteria." The following bacteria, all well-known enemies of modern science's war on bacterial infection, grew optimally on alkaline media of pH 7.4 and above: *staphylococcus* (staph infection), *streptococcus* (strep throat), *pneumococcus* (pneumonia), *h. influenza* (the flu), *meningococcus* (meningitis), *corymbacterium diptheriae* (diphtheria), *clostridium tetani* (tetanus), and others.

Dr. Jarvis wrote: "It becomes apparent, as one studies this list, that microorganisms harmful to the human body grow on an alkaline soil. This is particularly interesting in the light of the evidence that in dairy cows and human beings alike, an instinct exists which leads them to seek an acid intake. In the light of the above evidence, it seems reasonable to suspect that pathogenic bacteria which are harmful to the body are in the world for another purpose than to cause sickness in human beings. Nature has spread acid vegetation about with a lavish hand, apparently to prevent infestation of the body with pathogenic microorganisms, turning into infection of the body by these same microorganisms. The instinct leading animals and humans to seek acid vegetation and acid liquids has been given as a protection."

Informed of this, we can easily theorize why a high intake of ascorbic acid—even though neither Dr. Giorgi nor Dr. Lee considered it to be, of and by itself, functional vitamin C—is a popular and somewhat effective bacterial infection protector. It acidifies the body, creating an unfavorable medium of growth for pathogenic bacteria. But one should note that, acting in this way, ascorbic acid is not producing a "vitamin effect" but rather an acidifying effect. Apple cider vinegar is 5 percent *acetic acid*, a natural colorless crystalline acid normally found in the body. It is substantially less expense than ascorbic acid and does a better job at lower doses at acidifying the body. Two or three tablespoons of apple cider vinegar in some water, juice, or tea provide plenty of low-cost, pH-lowering acetic acid. If money is to be spent on vitamin C, it should be for the entire vitamin C spectrum or complex including the P or rutin factor.

So, as we see, the body uses the vitamins and minerals as a means of increasing the success of the immune response. Knowing this, it is easy to understand why the best way to help the immune system is to first cleanse the tissues and then fortify the body with natural whole complex nutrients.

NATURE'S CHEMISTRY OR MAN-MADE CHEMICALS

There can be little doubt that the greatest and most enduring of medical discoveries of the twentieth century were the vitamins. Here, at last, was the discovery of factors that *caused health*. Vitamin A (1912, the first vitamin to be discovered) was named *retinol* because, without it, a healthy retina in the eye could not be formed. Then it was found to cure night blindness. And that was just the beginning. Along came the B vitamins and the cures for beri-beri, pellagra, pernicious anemia, nerve degeneration, enlarged heart, energy production, and much more. These factors all came from unprocessed, whole, natural foods.

It was becoming increasingly clear that vitamins were biological complexes, bundles of enzymes and trace minerals, biological wheels within wheels within wheels. Trying to identify a vitamin in terms of a single chemical structure is self-defeating, because you have to have the whole complex to get the vitamin function. The failure of the pharmaceutical approach to vitamins originated in the chemists' synthetic isolation of a single element uncombined with its biological matrix. But the discovery of the vitamins coincided with the boom in industrial, agricultural, and pharmaceutical chemistry, which was crowding its way into all facets of life. But it was in the attempted duplication of living things, like artificial fertilizers or vitamins, that chemistry had its most distorting influence.

In his textbook on the new medical science of clinical ecology, *Human Ecology and Susceptibility to the Chemical Environment*, Seventh Edition, 1980, Theron G. Randolph, M.D., wrote, "A synthetically derived substance may cause a reaction in a chemically susceptible person when the same material of natural origin is tolerated, despite the two substances having identical chemical structures. This point is illustrated by the frequency of clinical reactions to synthetic vitamins—especially vitamins B_1 and C—when these naturally occurring vitamins are tolerated. There is also other evidence indicating that the biological activity of synthetic and natural vitamins is not identical."

The implications of this upon our general state of health are profound. The modern western diet has relied upon the process of "enrichment" of foods with synthetic vitamins, after they had been denuded of all or most naturally occurring nutrients through processing and refinement. As in the case of all *enriched flour* and *enriched rice* products, it is assumed that all you have to do to make these staple foods healthful is to spray a few synthetic vitamins back in. But, white bleached wheat flour has more than thirty known nutrients removed with four synthetically added back in. Enrichment of flour began in 1939 with a federal law.

It is more than interesting to observe that the first mention of "heart failure" by that name appeared in medical literature in 1912. Sudden death by heart attack was extremely rare during the last century as evidenced by a lack of a medical term for it. The first commercially milled and bleached flour process, in which the vitamin-containing germ (vitamins E and B complexes and trace minerals) and fiber-rich bran are removed, occurred in this country about 1905. One of Dr. Harvey Wiley's goals as first head of the Bureau of Chemistry, which is now the Food and Drug Administration (FDA), was to use the newly enacted Pure Food and Drug Law of 1906 to declare refined and bleached flour products an adulterated food, thereby preventing interstate shipment. He was undermined in his efforts by powerful commercial interests with strong political allies. By the early 1920s the epidemic of coronary heart attacks began in this country. It soon became clear, as vitamins and other nutrients were being discovered, that some protective factors in food were being stripped out. In 1939, the FDA required all wheat flour to be enriched with a few synthetic factors. They are: thiamin (B_1), riboflavin (B_2), nicotinic acid (B_3), and iron. Today, coronary heart disease kills over half of all American men and is the leading cause of death. A last note, here: The factors removed from flour by commercial milling are known as "millfeeds," and are fed to livestock which are raised for a profit.

However, adding artificial vitamins back into denuded grains and cereals is disgustingly profitable. Profits are wonderful, but they should be earned in an honorable way. The newsletter of The Center for Science in the Public Interest,

Nutrition Action (Vol. 16, No. 1), reports that the only difference between General Mills' Wheaties and Total cereals is that 1.5 cents' worth of synthetic vitamins are sprayed on Total. Total is then sold for 65 cents more than Wheaties. This practice alone has generated $425 million in additional profits since 1972 for General Mills.

It is not hard to understand why, when medical experiments are performed with synthetic vitamin fractions, these counterfeits fail to produce impressive results. But a reductionist mentality seeks to understand the whole by dismantling it to its parts. This precludes the wholistic principle that the whole is greater than the sum of its parts.

For example, what if we tried to understand the properties of water (H_2O) by testing hydrogen separately and oxygen separately. Presumably, we would learn enough about each to understand what their combined characteristics would be. Combined as two parts hydrogen and one part oxygen, H_2O will extinguish fire. It is water. Separately, the elements are among the most flammable and explosive elements in the universe. The functions are exactly the reverse in their isolated state from their organically combined state. Similarly, vitamins function as biological mechanisms only when whole and complete, combined with their synergists, as in whole food. Isolated into synthetic chemicals, they fail as catalysts. The only hope for a vitamin effect in our body from a synthetic is to recombine, once in the body, with synergistic factors that may be available. Often, the synergists are not freely available in the bloodstream. It is for this reason that most Americans merely *rent* their vitamin pills, and have the world's most expensive urine in the process. Vitamins are not meant to be eliminated in urine any more than silverware is to be thrown out with the leftovers.

J. I. Rodale, the American naturalist, wrote wisely on this subject in his classic work *The Complete Book of Food and Nutrition*. He wrote, "We *must* take vitamins if we wish to be healthy and the nation as a whole must do it, or God alone knows what will happen to the second or third generation coming up—generations inheriting weaknesses passed on to them by us, generations which few of us will live to see unless we augment our diet with vitamins and minerals. And, as parting advice, don't take coal tar [synthetic] vitamins. Examine every bottle. Be sure that the vitamins you take are extracted from food. Scientific research proves that this is best."

AN APPROACH TO HEALTH—NUTRITION OR APPLIED TOXICOLOGY?

When medical reports discuss nutritional supplements, invariably the assertion that vitamin and mineral supplements can be toxic comes up. It is usually not mentioned that unrealistic pharmacological dosages are needed to induce toxicity, and that natural food source supplements never come close to approaching those levels in recommended doses. Only synthetic vitamins approach these mega-levels in the name of "high potency". What is ironic about such expressed fears of toxic levels of nutrients by medical people is that toxicology itself is the cornerstone of their approach. This is no secret to anyone who understands modern medicine. A current example is *The Surgeon General's Report On Nutrition and Health, 1988*, which clearly spells this out: "All pharmacologic therapies induce side effects [pharmacology has been described as 'applied toxicology' because even the desirable effects of drugs are obtained by altering—poisoning normal metabolic function], and high-dose nutritional therapies are no exception." This quote has two startling revelations for the average layman. First, all drugs, as Royal Lee stated in a previous quote, are poisons, by definition. Second, abnormally high levels of isolated nutrients are not actually nutrients, but drugs. Only synthetic supplements achieve drug status.

BACK TO THE THYROID AND THE ENDOCRINE SYSTEM

The endocrine system and immune system are the most vitamin- and mineral-dependent systems. Our individual survival depends upon their health. There are several substances to be alert to that are potentially dangerous and poisonous to the glands. Sodium fluoride is one of them. In its natural state, fluorine is an essential trace mineral present in bones and teeth as fluoride, where it helps calcium make these tissues hard. That is *calcium fluoride* and is most often found naturally occurring in well water. What is added to municipal drinking waters is *sodium fluoride,* which is quite different from the natural calcium fluoride. Excessive doses can be very toxic, and by excessive we are speaking of minute doses to start with. Toxic levels have been shown at merely one part per million *(ppm).* Calcium is an antidote for sodium fluoride poisoning. You can fill a library with the literature from around the world about the negative effects of sodium fluoride. It has been cited as one of the most potentially toxic factors to the thyroid and endocrine system. You don't have to have a Ph.D. in chemistry to understand why.

This relates to enzymes, which relate, again, to plants. Considering all that vegetation manufactures for our planet, it is no wonder we honor it by calling our own factories "plants." Of all the substances produced by plants, the vitamin is its crowning glory. A vitamin has been described as a substance that will make you sick if you don't eat it! Sodium fluoride is a vitamin inhibitor. It is an enzyme inhibitor. Among scores of identified enzymes it inhibits, it can destroy the important bodily enzyme phosphatase, which is vital to the metabolism of vitamins. In other words, it can destroy the catalysts that make vitamins work.

Fluorine is a halogen molecule. The halogens form a distinct chemical group, including fluorine, chlorine, iodine, and bromine. This chemical group has the same electrical charge, all lacking one electron in their shell. As such, they combine easily with smaller molecules that have an extra electron. Of these halogens, fluorine and chlorine are two of the most potentially poisonous substances on the planet.

SUBSTITUTES CAN BE DANGEROUS TO DEADLY

One of the halogens, iodine, the trace element of the sea, represents about 65 percent by weight of the hormone thyroxin. This is the hormone that regulates metabolism, or the rate at which our bodies use energy. Parenthetically, Dr. Lee was the engineer who developed the first patent for making protein-bound iodine so that it doesn't burn your stomach when you take it as a supplement. Protein-bound iodine is found in sea-food such as kelp and dulse.

If you're deficient in protein-bound iodine, the body may try to make thyroxin out of the next closest material, which is what? Another available halogen molecule, sodium fluoride; available because it is added artificially to half of all public water systems in America. This potentially toxic material now concentrates in a very small gland in the body, the thyroid. Researchers in Finland recommended against fluoridation of their water after observing a 25 percent weight gain in three years in a sodium fluoride test on residents of a small village. A weakened thyroid from the medicated water was suspected for the weight gain. The body will utilize the materials closest to specifications. What a difference one mineral can make. Would you accept payment in lead instead of gold?

During the three years after the Chernobyl nuclear catastrophe in April 1986, cancer rates have doubled among residents of a contaminated farm region. There are Soviet newspaper reports of calves being born without heads and limbs. Radioactive iodine is often leaked into the atmosphere at such disasters. *Moscow News* reports that over 50 percent of the children in the Narodichsky region of the Ukraine have developed thyroid disease. The radioactive iodine will concentrate where? In the thyroid, doing irreparable damage to it. The Polish government issued iodine pills to the population immediately following the Chernobyl disaster.

I know people who have relatives in an area outside the Soviet Union affected by the Chernobyl disaster. Not long ago, with their soil and water contaminated by the drifting radioactive clouds and rain, they started losing their hair. These people called me and said, "What should we do?"

I thought for a moment. Then, as if Zeus put the words in my head and they came through my voice, I said loudly: *"Move! Don't Stay There! You Don't Live Where Nuclear Fallout Is Falling Out Of The Sky! Is This A Trick Question? We Have Nuclear Waste Sites In America; We Don't Put People There!"* Besides the ridiculousness of some people, I do understand, after all, that if I had to pack up and move and lose everything, it would be difficult. However, you have to put everything into perspective, and life comes first.

Protein-bound iodine is in fresh seafood and seaweed. I'm glad to see that people are eating more fish, and that's great. I don't want to upset you about what poisons are continuously dumped into the ocean and what's getting into the fish—the mercury, the agripoisons, and the spills from the oil industry. Hospital waste, illegally dumped in the oceans, washes up on the shore with blood-filled vials containing the AIDS virus, syringes, and other toxic debris. The ocean should be a source of perfection as it is our universal center of nutrition.

As we noted, you can contaminate the soil and you can deplete the soil, but you can never deplete the sea; you can only contaminate it. The sea is always whole and complete. But it is poisoned from man's dumping and agricultural run-off. DDT has been found in the livers of penguins in the South Pole. The Earth's oceans and winds are like our body's bloodstream and lymph system circulating throughout. So the pristine waters of the Arctic Ocean ultimately mingle with toxic agricultural runoff from some Illinois farm whose treated soil erodes into the Mississippi River, flows south to the Gulf of Mexico, and follows the Gulf Stream into the Atlantic Ocean and north throughout the world.

Protein-bound iodine is a very important radiation protective factor. If you have enough iodine, the body won't try to absorb the other halogen molecules, and will resist the radioactive iodine from a nuclear discharge. Chloride or chlorine is now added to virtually all the municipal water supplies as a method for sterilizing certain impurities. Non-chemical and safe alternatives are available for this task. But this is part of the cause of the current *Candida albicans* yeast infestation problem. Sterilizing the gut somewhat with a substance that is essentially Clorox every time we drink water out of the tap, just washing chlorine into the gut, sterilizing natural, healthy, friendly bacteria, allows *Candida albicans* to take over the gut. This isn't the only cause of *Candida*, but it's a chronic cause that's always present. A headline in the *Denver Post* in the summer of 1988 declared that Denver water was swimming in chlorine. "The drinking of chlorinated water has finally been officially linked to an increased incidence of colon cancer." This was the conclusion of an epidemiologist at Oak

Ridge Associated Universities, and reported in the April 1989 *Acres, USA.* The report concluded that drinking chlorinated water for fifteen years or more was conducive to an increased risk of colon cancer. The report added that bathing in chlorinated water, because of absorption through the skin, was equal to drinking two quarts of chlorinated water.

THE DARK SIDE OF FLUORIDE

The chemical cousin of chlorine is the halogen molecule fluorine, a widely distributed trace mineral of the Earth. But naturally occurring fluorine is a far cry from artificial fluoride, medicated into municipal drinking water of half the American population.

There are cities and communities that choose to fluoridate their water supply, for the usually stated reason of reducing dental caries. Proponents of fluoridation point to a 50 percent reduction in children's cavities in United States cities that artificially fluoridate. But have these communities known the real facts when deciding whether or not to fluoridate? *In the nonfluoridated cities across the United States there has been an equal reduction in children's cavities!* On August 1, 1988, the prestigious and authoritative trade journal *Chemical and Engineering News (C&EN),* the official weekly news organ of the 130,000-member American Chemical Society, reevaluated and reopened the entire debate on artificial fluoridation of public water supplies. It was an in-depth, balanced, and far-ranging examination of the issues involved. Responding to the *C&EN* fluoridation report, on August 23, 1988, the *Christian Science Monitor* printed an editorial reply entitled "Fluoridation Politics Makes Bad Science." According to this editorial, "There is growing awareness of one of the lesser-known scientific scandals—the suppression in the United States (and sometimes elsewhere) of research questioning fluoridation and *persecution of scientists who 'get out of line* [emphasis added].'" It likewise noted, "There is also continuing debate about the morality of imposing medication through the water supply." And, "Politicization of science is a public disgrace, placing propaganda above scientific objectivity." Organized opposition to debate the scientific merits of an idea or concept is more the style of a cult than a profession claiming to be the very standard of objectivity.

Nothing is more essential to protecting our good health than good water. We are physically 70 percent water. It purifies, nourishes, controls temperature, controls viscosity, and lubricates us. Where there is water, there is life. We consume it every day to live and can survive only a few days without it. Therefore, any issue about adding artificial substances to our most crucial commodity, water, should be the rightful concern of all citizens and scientists. The following are some relevant extracts from the *Chemical and Engineering News* August 1, 1988 report:

Valid basis for growing concern: *"Hundreds of papers [have been] published in reputable journals, a . . . large body of evidence of potential hazards."* (Page 27.)

Dental benefit claims questionable: *"Reductions in dental caries are just as great in nonfluoridated as in fluoridated areas."* (Page 30.)

Unsightly mottling of teeth: *"Several studies indicate . . . that the prevalence of dental fluorosis is rising, particularly at fluoride levels of 1 ppm."* (Page 33.)

Early stages of skeletal fluorosis: *"Doses as low as 2 to 5 milligrams per day [the amount of two to five liters of one ppm of fluoridated water] can cause the preclinical and early clinical stages."* (Page 35.) This is generally unrecognized in the United States because *"Most doctors in the U.S. . . . do not know how to diagnose it."* (Page 37.)

Osteoporosis and fluoride treatment: *"Well-designed studies have found no evidence of a beneficial effect [of fluoridation] on osteoporosis."* (Page 39.)

Hypersensitivity and side-effect reactions from fluoridated water: *"Dutch doctors performed double-blind experiments on patients who became ill after fluoridation began in the Netherlands [now banned]. By using coded bottles of drinking water, some fluoridated and some not, the physicians showed that the symptoms [e.g., muscular weakness, chronic fatigue, excessive thirst, headaches, skin rashes, joint pains, digestive upsets, tingling in extremities, and loss of mental acuity] were caused by fluoride, rather than some other factor."* (Pages 39–40.)

Enzymatic and mutagenic effects: Produced *"a transient decrease in human serum enzyme activity associated with the advent of water fluoridation."* (Page 40.) *"Tests . . . show sodium fluoride mutagenic for cultured lymphoma cells."* (Page 41.)

Birth defects and cancer: There was *"a higher rate of Down's syndrome births among mothers in fluoridated areas."* (Page 41.) *"After correcting for age, race, and sex, the death rate from cancer of the digestive system was 9% higher with fluoridated water."* (Page 42.)

Finally, and most depressing of all, come the *C&EN* revelations of an ongoing, decades-old organized suppression of scientific papers and research by competent scientists who cast any doubt on the questionable benefits or present possible dangers of medicating public water with artificial fluoride. This stratagem to asphyxiate honest scientific debate, rather than an isolated case relating to this subject, appears to form a consistent pattern of commercial interests elevated above public health since the day Dr. Harvey Wiley was removed from office in 1912. The following quotes from the *C&EN* report speak of a pseudo-science that defends its established paradigm by casting personal attacks and defamation on those (including peers) presenting differing scientific views rather than discussing, debating, or researching the actual merits of the various scientific findings presented. Resorting to this style of character assassination action would seem to be a virtual admission of standing on scientifically wobbly ground.

"If the lifeblood of science is open debate of evidence, scientific journals are the veins and arteries of the body scientific. Yet journal editors often have refused for political reasons to publish information that raises questions about fluoridation." (Page 36.)

"Dogmatic assertions and attacks on the credibility of the opposi-tion." (Pages 28–29.) *[In ethical science, no one should be perceived as "opposition" if the aim is to ascertain the truth of the matter. Un-derstandably, differences will arise through interpretation of unbiased research and should be clarified through open and vigorous debate and duplication of experimental results.]*

"Ever since the Public Health Service (PHS) endorsed fluorida-tion in 1950, detractors have charged that PHS and the medical and dental establishment, such as the American Medical Association (AMA) and the American Dental Association (ADA), have sup-pressed adverse scientific information about its effects.

"Some of those who generally support fluoridation make similar charges . . . [an editor of the Academy of General Dentistry wrote that] . . . "supporters of fluoridation have had an 'unwillingness to release any information that would cast fluorides in a negative light,'" and that organized dentistry has lost "its objectivity—the ability to consider varying viewpoints together with scientific data to reach a sensible conclusion." (Page 36.)

EPA scientist Robert J. Carton stated that the agency "omits 90% of the literature on mutagenicity, most of which suggests fluoride is a mutagen." (Page 36.)

"Most authoritative scientific overviews of fluoridation have omit-ted negative information about it, even when the oversight is pointed out." C&EN *cites as an example of this a professor of environmental medicine in Denmark, Phillipe Grandjean, writing about a WHO study on fluorides stating, "Information which could cast any doubt on the advantage of fluoride supplements was left out by the Task Group. Unless I had been present myself, I would have found it hard to believe."* (Page 36.)

"In 1982, John A. Colquhoun, former principal dental officer in the Department of Health in Auckland, New Zealand, was told after writing a report that showed no benefit from fluoridation in New Zealand the department refused him permission to publish it." (Page 36.)

"ADA and PHS also have actively discouraged research into the health risks of fluoridation by attacking the work or the character of

the investigators. As part of their political campaign, they have over the years collected information on perceived antifluoridation scientists, leaders, and organizations. . . . It is used not only in efforts to counteract arguments of the antifluoridationists, but also to discredit the work and objectivity of U.S. scientists whose research suggests possible health risks from fluoridation." (Page 37.)

"Consumer advocate Ralph Nader calls it [false intelligence reports and a smear campaign to personally demean anyone of opposing view] 'an institutionalized witch hunt.'"

The facts and arguments for or against fluoridation, expressed in the *C&EN* news report, should be read and studied by every concerned person. Reprints of the *C&EN* special report are available for five dollars (three dollars for five or more copies) from: *C&EN*, Distribution, Room 210, 1155–16th St., NW, Washington, DC 20036.

Dr. Royal Lee and the Lee Foundation for Nutritional Research were perhaps the first informed and vigorous opponents to fluoridation. Lee called it "an attempt to treat a deficiency disease [dental caries], a case of starvation, with a poisonous drug."

Do you know where the fluoride comes from that's put into municipal water? For the most part, fluoride is a highly toxic by-product of aluminum production. The aluminum industry, after mining and processing bauxite, has nowhere to dump all this toxic waste. Fluoride is also a by-product of phosphate fertilizer manufacturing. After some research, they finally concluded that they could make a case for putting it in public drinking water, got the dentists behind it to push it, and before too long, without long-term scientific studies, we had fluoridation of most public water supplies. Although it was once legal, fluoridation is now banned throughout most of Europe and Japan. Of considerable significance in the banning of fluoridation in Denmark, was the public outrage of forced medication of the public water. Interestingly, those same countries are ranked ahead of the United States in national health ratings made by the WHO. I personally doubt that fluoridation of the water supply was a Communist plot, as some have suggested. If it was not, however, someone in the KGB in charge of this kind of thing should have been fired for overlooking a great opportunity. Since 15 percent of the Soviet drinking water is fluoridated, perhaps it was an Afghani plot!

We have come to understand that the body will always use the natural before it will try to substitute the counterfeit. Of course, the body must attempt to use what's available; it will do the best it can. People have eaten shoe leather to stay alive. They've eaten rats. But the body doesn't want to do that. It will always take the high-quality choice first.

THE HUMAN BODY MUST MAKE CHOICES

Protecting the body from radiation with protein-bound iodine is critical. However, don't depend on the iodine put in iodized salt. This is an inferior, less-usable form, just barely enough to prevent overt goiter. It is minimal protection to the thyroid. Harvests from the sea are the best.

For the most part, H-bomb testing above ground, is not done anymore—unless it's a seemingly unimportant section of the planet such as the South Pacific, near Tahiti and Fiji, where the French and South Africans do their above-ground nuclear testing.

Those innocent native people just get zapped. After all, to the world's nuclear nations, they're not part of the economic scheme of things. Those areas seem to be the last region in the world to still suffer above-ground nuclear testing. That's why the courageous crew on the Greenpeace ship was sabotaged by the French secret service in a New Zealand harbor, because that Greenpeace ship always planted itself near ground-zero in the South Pacific ocean to block the tests. People wonder who the real heroes of today are. They are the people who are working at gut core levels to keep life on this planet.

What scientists have found is that strontium-90 from nuclear fallout ends up causing bone cancer. It gets into the grass, and the cows eat the grass. Then it's in their milk, and you drink the milk, eat the butter, eat the cheese, eat the yogurt, and you absorb the strontium-90. What does strontium-90 look like to the human body? Calcium. For all the body's understanding of all the many forms in which minerals can appear, strontium-90 looks like calcium. To protect against strontium-90 poisoning, take large amounts of ionizable forms of calcium, such as calcium lactate. Some confuse the word "lactate" with the word for milk sugar, "lactose." A lactate form simply means bound with lactic acid, a natural digestive product.

Since the dairy industry started pasteurizing the milk earlier this century, we've lost our best source of ionizable calcium in the diet. Ionizable calcium is the most absorbable, usable, free form of calcium that can be drawn into all bones and tissues in the body. In the healthy body, calcium is more abundant than all the other minerals added together. There is always a great demand for calcium. But, like the proper currency in the right country, it must be in the correct form to use.

When the dairy industry started pasteurizing the milk, they made calcium absorption and utilization more difficult. You have to ask yourself, why do we have a nation that has more osteoarthritis, osteoporosis, arteriosclerosis, kidney stones, and cataracts—all the calcium-related degenerative diseases—than any other country, when we have more dairy products than any nation in history? I have never seen a response to the issue of the *nutritional* inferiority of sterilized milk from any industry scientist. From dairy products, we may potentially have a greater source of calcium, but it's in a less available form. It's pasteurized, heat-sterilized, and it has become a cooked food at that point. When you cook nature's perfect raw food, chemically altering it, it becomes difficult to digest and assimilate. The resulting deficiency helps to create a greater vulnerability to strontium-90 poisoning.

Because strontium-90 looks like the molecular structure of calcium to the body, the body absorbs it, thinking. "Oh, here's a real concentrated source of calcium; I need this in the bones."

Strontium-90 gets into the bones and just burns the bone marrow into mutant cancer cells, as it irradiates the bones. Whenever you know about any strontium-90 exposure or nuclear above-ground testing, you should always make sure you have plenty of ionizable calcium in your diet. You want to build up your reserves of ionizable calcium so that the body won't absorb that strontium-90 and it will pass right out the gut. The body is now satiated with ionizable calcium, the preferred form of the mineral when available.

You see what I mean by a broader context of the immune system. It's not just fighting AIDS, it's realizing that we are destroying the immune fabric, the armor, of the whole eco-system/food chain resulting in a personal assault of our well-being across a wide spectrum. Calcium is critical for prevention of strontium-90 poisoning from radioactive fallout, just as protein-bound iodine is essential for protection against radioactive iodine from accidents at nuclear power plants.

WHAT ABOUT SKIN CANCER AND SUNSHINE?

Let's consider some more about the implications of the ozone layer depletion, introduced in the previous chapter. Malignant melanoma is up 80 percent in recent decades. "Well," you say, "That's okay. I'll just go out and buy some sunscreen." In Philadelphia, Jefferson Medical College researchers report that sunscreens above sun protection factor 8 (SPF 8) can cause vitamin deficiency by blocking vitamin D production in the skin (I've seen SPFs above 30). But, as an answer, is our consciousness that shallow? Does that mean that all the Aborigines in Australia for instance, who live outdoors, will get melanoma and die because they don't have sunscreen? We are a tired race, weary of fighting the effects of our insane causing.

The problem here is, we've torn holes in our own ozone layer—a good symbol of our current consciousness. One of the things to keep in mind is that to keep the flesh from becoming totally susceptible to the effects of ultraviolet radiation, the skin needs to be strong and hard. Skin is our body's most outer defense.

For example, we wouldn't cook over an open flame with a plastic pot. Why? Because it would melt. But we would cook with steel because steel won't melt. I'm using a crude analogy to make the point that when you apply heat to something that's strong, damage is resisted.

People have so little strength in their skin because of their vitamin, fatty acid, and mineral deficiencies—which go all the way back to the soil, which goes back to where we started. There are so few trace elements in the demineralized soil, the skin of the Earth, that likewise the skin of the people who live upon it is made even more susceptible to the effect of ultraviolet light. We will expand on this after we lay some groundwork in the next section.

THE IMPORTANT RELATIONSHIP BETWEEN VITAMINS AND MINERALS

Dr. John Miller, from Chicago, was one of the greatest mineral metabolism experts in the world. He was a leader in developing chelated mineral supplements. This significantly enhanced the delivery of the mineral across the gut barrier into the bloodstream. A chelated mineral, as mentioned, is one that is bound to amino acids. As the amino acid is easily absorbed, the heavier mineral "hitchhikes" a ride through the intestinal wall into the bloodstream.

Dr. Lee built on much of Dr. Miller's work on minerals. In his studies on calcium, Dr. Miller found that the vitamin that controlled calcium absorption into the blood had a natural antagonist, unofficially called vitamin F. What vitamin do we get from the sun? Vitamin D. It is important to understand the relationship between vitamins and minerals because they are entirely different substances.

Let me illustrate: intellectually, for the sake of this discussion, you could classify minerals as being dumb. As much as I love them, and I can't live without them, minerals obey one primary physical law: *gravity*. Minerals, in this way, are alive and they're beautiful, but they're dumb. Vitamins, on the other hand, are, compared with minerals, very intelligent. Vitamins help control the flow of minerals through the body. Vitamins help the metabolism and utilization of minerals.

We speak of rickets as a deficiency disease that involves deformity of the bones caused by poor absorption of calcium into the bones. Then, why don't we call rickets a calcium-deficiency disease? It's because we call it a vitamin D deficiency disease! It's not vitamin D that's making the bones bow, it's the lack of calcium. Fortunately, the discoverers of this knew not to blame poor calcium; it didn't know any better. Calcium cannot get through the gut and into the bloodstream without vitamin D.

Once in the blood, calcium must then be delivered to the tissues, and here is the problem: In every single heat-and-sun-related disorder—sunstroke, heat prostration, hyperthermia, fever—you'll always find elevated blood calcium levels. When heat is a factor, you'll find that the calcium levels in the blood will be unusually high. In this regard, Dr. Lee pointed out that this is one of the main functions of a fever—to pull ionizable calcium out of the bones and draw it into the blood where it is useful fighting the infection. The fever is a defensive adaptation during infection, because there's a deficiency of available ionizable calcium. The body will burn a high fever to free calcium from the bone, grab that calcium (which draws out in the heat) and then transport it through the blood to fight against an infection in the respiratory tract or wherever. If you turn off the fever, as most mothers rush to do with aspirin, you block the body's correct biological response.

CALCIUM CONTROL, SUNBURN, AND YOUR SKIN

What makes vitamin D potentially toxic (hypervitaminosis D) is that it is capable of elevating the blood calcium level so high that blood viscosity becomes dangerously high, laden with heavy calcium molecules. The bone-building mineral, calcium, in excessive amounts, can thicken the blood and reduce capillary circulation. The reason calcium is in the blood, as with most nutrients, is for transportation. Just as the automobile is not our destination, we enter it to get where we are going. The reason we have a bloodstream is to transport and deliver things.

Vitamin F, which we know consists of essential polyunsaturated fatty acids (linolenic, linoleic, and arachidonic acid), ionizes the calcium to transport it *out* of the blood and *into* the tissue. This was Dr. Miller's great contribution in understanding calcium metabolism.

Dr. Miller showed that this antagonist of vitamin D, vitamin F, transported calcium by means of attaching an extra electron to the calcium molecule. One effect of that electron is that the calcium molecules become polarized and lined up in the exact same direction. This could be likened to a pile of iron filings; if you wave a magnet over the iron filings, they all respond to the magnetic force and line up in the same direction.

When the vitamin F complex is in the blood, it ionizes and polarizes the calcium molecules, then the calcium begins to flow out of the blood into the tissue. Vitamin D deionizes calcium; vitamin F ionizes it. This results in decreased blood calcium and increased tissue calcium.

Most people have limited amounts of ionizable calcium in the body because they depend upon pasteurized dairy foods for their calcium. Then, when they take a vitamin D supplement (which is unnecessarily synthetically fortified into most processed, pasteurized, and homogenized milk) or go out into the sun, which is for all practical purposes a vitamin D supplement, their blood calcium levels build up. But the calcium has no means of being drawn into the skin. The skin, very deficient in calcium, has lost its hardest mineral protection against the sun.

Calcium isn't just for the bones; calcium adds to every tissue exactly what it adds to the bone: strength and structure. Calcium adds strength and structure to every cell in the body, particularly the skin, which is the largest organ of the human body. The skin is a big user of calcium. Thus, if you're eating margarine; if you're eating oleo products, hydrogenated oil products; if you're cooking the life out of your oils; you're not getting vitamin F factors. Then, even if you have calcium, you're not going to put it into the skin to protect the skin against solar radiation.

CAN YOU TAKE THE HEAT?

We've cut this hole in the immune system of the atmosphere (the ozone layer); we're increasingly exposed to higher levels of ultraviolet (UV) rays, which means that if you're cooking at 350°F, maybe you'll get by with stainless steel. If you could cook at 1,200°F, you would need titanium-coated steel. Supersonic jets get a titanium skin. The point is that if we're increasingly exposed to higher levels of radiation, we need a harder protective surface.

Oftentimes, muscle cramps fail to respond to calcium supplements, and for good reason. You may have a muscle cramp, so you take calcium, but it doesn't work. Therefore, you must not have a calcium deficiency, right? Wrong. You probably do have enough calcium in your body, but the preponderance of it is in the blood. Dr. Royal Lee called this "tissue calcium starvation." What you were deficient in was the vitamin F that would transport calcium from the blood into the tissue.

NOT ALL FORMS OF CALCIUM ARE ASSIMILATED

A first-year student in biochemistry should know that you cannot absorb calcium in an alkaline medium; it turns hard, crystallizes, and can't get through the gut wall. You need calcium in soft, organic form. The acid of the stomach takes calcium and breaks it down by washing it in hydrochloric acid (HCl). Anything washed in HCl tends to become soft. Then it goes into the duodenum where, in the upper gastrointestinal (GI) tract, calcium is absorbed into the blood.

But if you take an antacid, it matters little how much calcium it has; the de-acidifying action of it is going to deter absorption of the calcium. Remember this: The stomach and the GI tract are technically not considered to be inside the body. Am I anatomically correct? That's right, the gut is anatomically outside the body. The calcium in an antacid rarely gets into the body, because it stays in the gut, and remains undelivered to the bloodstream. The claims of Madison Avenue's advertising whizzes have people convinced otherwise.

Your gut doesn't need the calcium; your body tissues do. So this whole calcium-in-antacids nonsense is another example of television advertising managers' practicing medicine without a brain.

7
Detoxification, Strengthening, and Renewal

Before you fortify, first detoxify. How do you know if you need to go on a cleansing program? In this country, virtually everyone needs it to some degree. How can you avoid it? It's nothing against your character or your personality. It's not as if you're unclean, *unkosher*. If you live on Earth in the 1980s, you qualify for a detoxification program.

Here's another point to keep in mind. Don't think of detoxification as a single, therapeutic remedy: *"Oh yes, I did that, I went on a fast eight years ago. It was excellent. I felt great."* Detoxification needs incorporation into our lifestyle.

It may initially, or now and again, have to take a certain overt form, such as a fast, colonics, or other methods of overt purgings. However, our lifestyle needs to be a very low-residue, non-toxic type of lifestyle that is, in a sense, an on-going, cleansing lifestyle.

WHO SHOULD BE FIRST IN LINE FOR DETOXIFICATION?

How do you identify the individual in need of detoxification? Unless most health professionals change their style of practice, they are not going to be in touch with the needs of a generally toxic patient. They can't simply say, "Well, I'm going to treat everyone this way." They are rarely trained in this work. Since the advent of the age of medical specialization, as soon as a symptom appears in some area, the patient is shuffled off to the specialist in charge of that fraction of the body. Who is taking a look at the totality of the patient? Could it be we have so many different diseases (22,000 listed) because we have so many different specialties? Nevertheless, one of the first clues of toxicity is multiple-system symptoms.

When the body is toxic, the bloodstream is toxic, the lymphatic system is toxic, thus the toxins circulate. The blood goes everywhere in the body, and the lymph travels throughout the body. When you have headaches, chronic indigestion and nausea, migrating joint pains and aches, and depression, that could well be toxicity. When you determine a person's symptoms and he says, "This isn't a survey of symptoms, this is my autobiography," you have a person who generally qualifies for detoxification.

Most doctors would love to be able to say, "We've just done a complete analysis on you, and every single problem you have is in the stomach." Oh, that would be great! Doctors should have nothing but patients like that all day. But they don't. They find these integrated disorders with multiple-system symptoms.

YOU CAN'T PUT OUT A FIRE BY BLOWING OUT THE SMOKE

Picture a building on fire. When the firemen arrive at a burning building, they might see smoke pouring out of twenty different windows. Can you imagine what would happen if the firemen treated the symptoms? They'd do more damage than the fire. They'd come in there with their axes and their hoses and their hooks and ladders and their water bombs, and they'd wreck the place. They'd put those hoses on every single window.

The smoke could be pouring through all the windows, but the fire may just be a little trash fire in some corner office. Still, the smoke goes everywhere. Likewise, in this way, toxicity often camouflages itself by circulating symptom-causing toxins throughout the body.

If you're harboring an infection in the spleen (the largest lymphatic organ), which is more common than generally thought, and the spleen is toxic with pus and lymph all backed up, then the spleen is not recycling useful parts of dying red blood cells, and it's not creating immunity-building antibodies. Soon there's a general depression in the body. You feel sick all over and you say, "I have a headache and I'm nauseated, and I'm always coming down with colds." Meanwhile, although the "fire" is in the spleen, the symptoms go everywhere. What's an important part of the answer? Cleanse.

Many of the side effects of detoxification, should they occur, are the same symptoms as toxicity: headaches, nausea, depression. As you release the waste, you're moving through a highly active transition. It can be uncomfortable for a short period.

Detoxification is a relatively aggressive process. Remember the symptoms of the flu? So, as the saying goes, "You can pay me now, or pay me later." The meaning here is that if you wait for a severe cold or flu to detoxify you, you will suffer more. You can modify the severity of a cleanse, depending on how you go about it. When you starve poisons out of your system, that's fairly aggressive. You don't want to detoxify faster than you can eliminate. The last thing you want to do is be on a detox program while constipated.

Health professionals should guide the detoxification process and have a big responsibility here: Not fearing a symptom that nature produces. While side effects from medical drugs signal reaction to a poison, side effects from natural healing are usually good signs. In fact, reactions to natural substances can reveal very useful information.

For example when somebody says, "That calcium just made me sick," you can usually say, "Oh, excellent; now we know you are most likely hypochlorhydric (low HCl levels in the stomach). This is great information that reveals a possible mineral absorption problem." Or, if someone says, "That fat-soluble chlorophyll supplement made me nauseated," you can usually say, "Great! How else would I have known that you didn't produce enough bile and it flows sluggishly out of your gall bladder? Now we know that fat-soluble vitamins and essential fatty acids are not being broken down properly." When you're using natural healing methods, every process is information: it's all part of the healing process. You aren't afraid of symptoms; you look for them. They're like the warning gauges on your car's dashboard. You would not think of covering them up so that you wouldn't receive annoying information that would require an intelligent response. Symptoms help guide us into the clear.

A WORD TO THE WISE

Before you spend money on expensive and exotic herbs and nutritional supplements to try to fortify your immune system, don't try to fortify on top of a toxic system. You would not pour new topsoil over a toxic waste sight and say that now it's okay to plant. Nor, after driving your car 10,000 miles since your last oil change, would it be wise to add clean, fresh oil. It would become instantly contaminated by the old, dirty oil. You would first drain your dirty oil. So, why take expensive nutritional supplements that are only going to go into a toxic system? Cleanse first, fortify second. Then, during the fortification, be consistent in a detoxifying lifestyle with the right variety of certified organically grown foods, and you will be as healthy as is possible, given the limitations of the world that we've created.

A complete detoxification program would aspire to accomplish the following: Normalize stomach pH; aid pancreatic enzyme production; flush gall bladder and thin the bile; de-fat and decongest the liver; build intestinal micro-flora; flush mucus and waste from the intestinal wall to free villi action and nutrient absorption; remove impacted colon fecal waste; stimulate peristaltic action for elimination; purify and build the blood; cleanse urinary tract and promote fluid balance;

promote lymphatic drainage; open skin pores; expectorate mucus from lungs; and open respiratory passageways. It could take from one to twelve months to accomplish this depending upon the individual. Your body knows.

Detoxification of the body will have profoundly positive effects on the mind. A British Government study reported in the English medical journal *The Lancet,* on January 14, 1989, that risk of getting Alzheimer's disease was 50 percent greater in areas with elevated levels of aluminum in the water. Cleansing the body of toxic metals such as aluminum must be seen as a primary goal in treating physical and mental disorders. Although this is a very recent finding, naturalist doctors have adamantly opposed human exposure to aluminum (such as cooking utensils) for fifty years. I knew one old osteopath from Texas who worked his way through osteopathic college in the 1930s by selling aluminum cookware. By the 1960s he was so convinced of the aluminum problem that he was overcome with guilt about all the pots and pans he had sold. He dug through every old record he could find, going through old drawers and digging through attic trash to reassemble a mailing list of his old customers from thirty years back. He then sent out a letter to all of them, urging them to throw away any remaining utensils he sold them. He explained what he had learned since his early days. Predictably, most of the letters came back unopened, but he did his best to undo his guileless error. In a few instances, some did write back saying they too had heard warnings and had thrown the cookware away many years before.

IT ISN'T WHO YOU KNOW, IT'S WHAT YOU KNOW

If you think the information in this book is rare and these insights of Dr. Lee and others that Dr. Jensen has offered for over sixty years are gems, it is very important to understand how you can apply this in your life so you can be well. Don't be fooled into thinking, "Only the rich know this." I used to be suspicious and think that. I used to think, "The rich know all this. They just don't want the masses to have access to it." I was wrong.

Do you remember *Tevye*, the lead character in *Fiddler on the Roof*, the big Jewish peasant who's in the barn singing the song, "If I Were A Rich Man"? He is rationalizing out loud why it would be good if God made him rich. He confesses that if he were a rich man, at last he would be respected by others, because, he says, "When you're rich, they think you really know." He was right—they *think* you really know. But, of course, you don't.

That is why Henry Ford II, one of the wealthiest men who ever walked the planet, died of iatrogenic causes from something as simple as respiratory distress in a hospital his father built. At the press conference following his death, his own physician said he died of complications caused by the lung machine he was placed on; this apparently created too much stress on his kidneys. The drugs they subsequently gave him to deal with this complication left his lungs open to infection, and with his immune system thus weakened, he soon died of pneumonia. All his money couldn't buy him a little knowledge of how to deal with respiratory distress—a man of only seventy years. He didn't know; his doctors didn't know. Don't think that when you're rich you really know. When it comes to ignorance of the laws of health, people are all tarred with the same brush.

YOUR MIND IS PART OF THE IMMUNE SYSTEM

Whenever you read nutrition or natural farming books, use great discernment in terms of how you want to apply the information. Be alert and use common sense. That's part of your immune system, too. Part of your immune system is your mind, not the judging mind, but the reasoning mind; the mind that can reason through choices and understand how to apply knowledge and where it fits is part of the immune system. Malnutrition and sickness weaken the mind and the mental aspect of the immune system.

Our spirit and feeling, our very instincts, are parts of the immune system as well. Civilization tends to dull instincts. The spirit tells the mind when something is on track. That inner voice we sometimes listen to will say, "It's okay to take more of this, it's okay to listen to more of this. This rings true." The spirit is part of the immune system. This is what I mean by the larger scope of the immune system.

Moreover, it's necessary to educate the mind so your choices and discernment can be wise. For example, I believe, based upon what I have learned, that it's terribly important that you try to get as high a percentage of organically grown food as you can in your diet. You see, not only are organically grown foods free of toxic chemicals, but the soil on which they grew must have been naturally healthy enough to allow sufficient immunity to survive insects and fungus. The organically grown food will contain substances worthy of being eaten. I think our values change when we realize that good food is worth paying for. Values are part of an acquired appreciation for what we have learned.

Dr. Bernard Jensen has said to me, "You've got to do the best you can with the circumstances at hand," and that's been good advice. Certainly, given the state of the world, we know our nutrition is always going to be sub-optimal. Where you have a choice, don't just consider money when it comes to buying chemical-free, organically grown food. If you have to pay two dollars a pound for certified organically grown grapes, versus sixty-nine cents a pound for sprayed grapes, let me point something out: It's better to pay a lot for something than a little for nothing. You're always ripped off no matter how little you pay for nothing. This is an economic fact.

Paying a fair price for clean, healthy, organically grown produce gives the organic grower what he deserves and keeps the honest soil-based (versus oil-based) farmer on the land. Support the guy who knows that good soil is what makes good food. This is what brings our mother, the Earth, into our bodies. Our mother still feeds us long after we go off the breast. Don't hesitate to pay top dollar when investing in the food your body is made from. *Depositing blank checks in our savings accounts will not bring us wealth any more than eating an empty harvest will bring our bodies health.*

I drive past at least five large commercial grocery stores on my way to the only place I shop locally. I know the grocer. I know his integrity. I know his concern. He does not allow irradiated foods or herbs in his store. Irradiation of foods, a preservation technique of exposing foods to high doses of radioactive material, has been banned in England since 1968 because of the disapproval by the British Medical Association regarding the technology. Perhaps the United States nuclear industry, desperate to get rid of cesium-125, a nuclear waste product, tore a page out of the aluminum industry's method for getting rid of their waste product, fluoride. But consumer resistance, the ultimate judge of any product, has, for now, slowed the introduction of irradiated produce and meat.

My grocer seeks out and develops connections with organic producers. He knows that people will support him by paying more for superior food. I'd rather have the spot on the apple than eat wax and pesticides. As Joni Mitchell sang, "Give me spots on my apples, save me the birds and the bees."

The best publication I know of to keep you up to date on organic agriculture is *Acres, USA,* published in Kansas City, Missouri. The founder and editor, Charles Walters, Jr., has set up a computer bulletin board whereby, with the use of a personal computer and modem, organic producers and sellers can meet each other and arrange costs and shipments for their produce. This is a great service that you can tell your local health food market or co-op about.

So, educate yourself about natural food and soil, and drive across town to pass up several chain-store supermarkets in support of the organic grower, and your own health. The only way a vote counts in this country is if it is cast with your dollar. Would you rather support the family farm or a billion dollar conglomerate? It's an important value judgment we have to make. Then you don't have to spend money on dandruff shampoos, acne creams, fluoridated toothpaste, and all the other "deficiency accessories" generally put in the grocery bag. Remember this simple rhyme: "The whiter the bread, the sooner you're dead."

A FABLE FOR OUR TIME

There once was a little bird that decided not to fly south with its flock in the autumn. Everything was so nice and colorful that he told his friends to leave without him. In a few weeks, the north wind began to blow, and sleet and snow began to fall. The little bird tried desperately to fly south, but his wings iced up and he crash-landed next to a barn. Just when he was about to freeze to death, a cow happened by and dropped a pile of manure on him. Pretty soon the warm manure thawed him out, and he felt so good he began to chirp. A cat in the barn came to check out the chirping, discovered the little bird, and ate him.

This story has three morals. First, everyone who drops a pile of manure on your head is not necessarily your enemy. Second, everyone who gets you out of a pile of manure is not necessarily your friend. Third, if you are warm and happy in a pile of manure, keep your mouth shut.

It would appear that the vast majority of the citizens of the industrialized world are warm and happy in the environmental equivalent of a pile of manure, and they're keeping their mouths shut. The ersatz comfort of modern "living" tends to desensitize people and hold them in a lethargic state. It might be noted that it is easier to control them in this state. Just as surely as their thermostat on the wall keeps their climate artificially tuned, the hollow food grown on empty soil keeps their bodies and minds dull, unproductive in manufacturing the chemical compounds of the brain and endocrine system. To once again quote Surgeon General Parran, *"Many well-to-do Americans who can eat what they like are so badly fed as to be physically inferior and mentally dull."*

Enfeebled as such, in this disconnected life, people actually don't want to know what is happening in reality, so they safely read about unreality in supermarket tabloids and popular magazines, which, no matter how outrageous the stories, require no response or action on their parts. They gulp their sugared pop and nibble their hydrogenated chips, oblivious to the garbage and radiation that infiltrates their water, their air, their soil. Pathetically, their biggest fear is "losing it all." Afraid of dying, the fear of truly living is greater.

The feeling seems to be, "There is only so much of the 'good life,' not everyone can have it, and I am lucky to have my share. I don't know Mother Earth, but I'll rest my soul in the bosom of Mother General Mills, or Mother Exxon, or

Mother Squibb, or Mother Del Monte, or Mother Du Pont, or Mother Safeway." Of course, loyalty to these "mothers" is as deep as a paycheck or discount coupon.

It's not life's design that there should be scarcity and deficiency. A look at a single human cell reveals a scientific wonder of biochemical dynamism, of manufacture and transportation, of efficient operation and abundant energy production, and of perfect waste management. As humans, we are composed of more than 100 trillion of these extraordinary, life-teeming cells. As wondrous and powerful as these cells are, it would seem that, as humans and a society, we have experienced less than the sum of our own parts.

We want *prosperity*, but that word should truly mean "prospirit." Wherever there's poverty, deficiency, and disease, there is a broken spirit. The prosperity of the land—or lack of it—reflects the spirit of the people, their healing, and their consciousness.

I repeat here from Chapter Two, "Our individual immune systems are inescapably linked to the planet Earth, of whose substance we are made." I hope that from what I have presented here, you can fathom my message. More than 2,700 years ago, the Hebrew prophet Isaiah expressed his vision of the last days of life on Earth. He saw the depleted, demineralized soil and the air pollution. He declared, "For the heavens shall vanish away like smoke [*he had no word for smog*], and the earth shall wax old like a garment [*threadbare of the material that binds it*], and they that dwell therein shall die in like manner [*the inhabitants would die in the same condition the Earth was in, demineralized like a worn-out garment*]." Is. 51:6

Though the call is not to go back to the Native Americans' way of life, we must nonetheless understand the wisdom of how these original ecologists allowed for integration and care for the land (forests, soils, grasslands, and waters) to be so excellent that ships bringing masses poured over here from Europe, Asia, and Africa. The wisdom of living ecologists had maintained the land in sustainable harmony.

Ultimately, we are "human" beings, i.e., "*humus*"—soil beings. Made of the Earth, we have the inherent strength, beauty, and dignity of the Earth in us. Look at our planet from outer space, marvel at its beauty; then remember, "I am made of that." When we act to protect the Earth, we respond to the deepest and most God-loving instinct in us. Suppress that, and we turn our backs on our own Mother. It is no sacrifice to save our Mother. All our health and longevity derives from the Earth, her substance and energy, and not the artificial "cures" of those who tread heavily upon her.

Answers are known, and they're available. If we move swiftly with a single purpose, we can restore the planet and ourselves. The planet needs healthy, strong souls who are going to be able to steer this sick and dying ship back in the right direction. To do this, we must begin with ourselves and align our values accordingly.

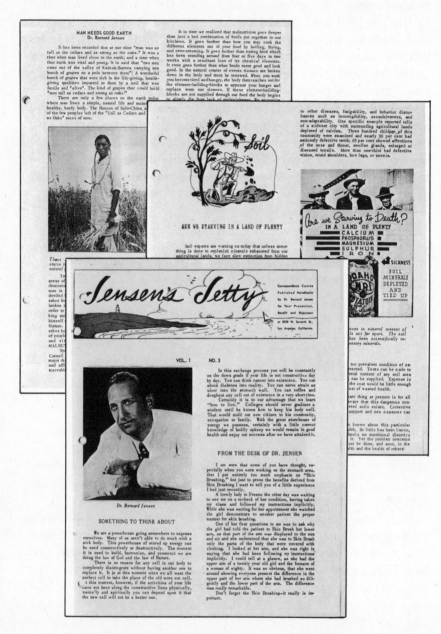

MAN NEEDS GOOD EARTH
Dr. Bernard Jensen

It has been recorded that at one time "man was as tall as the cedars and as strong as the oaks." It was a time when man lived close to the earth; and a time when that earth was vital and young. It is said that "two men came out of the valley of Kadesh-Barnea carrying one bunch of grapes on a pole between them"! A wonderful bunch of grapes that were rich in the life-giving, health-giving qualities imparted to them by a soil that was fertile and "alive". The kind of grapes that could build "men tall as cedars and strong as oaks!"

There are only a few places on the earth today where man lives a simple, natural life and maintains a healthy, hardy body. The Hunzas of Indo-China are of the few peoples left of the "Tall as Cedars and as Oaks" races of men.

It is time we realized that malnutrition goes deeper than just a bad combination of foods put together in our kitchens. It goes further than how you may cook the different elements out of your food by boiling, frying, and over-steaming. It goes further than eating food which has been standing around from four or five days to two weeks with a resultant loss of its chemical elements. It even goes further than what foods taste good and look good. In the natural course of events tissues are broken down in the body and must be renewed. When you work you become tired and hungry, the body then reaches out for the element-building-blocks to appease your hunger and replace worn out tissues. If these element-building-blocks are not supplied through our food the body begins to slowly die from lack of replenishment. We recognize

to other diseases, fatigability, and behavior disturbances such as incorrigibility, assaultiveness, and non-adaptability. One specific example reported tells of a midwest city with surrounding agricultural lands depleted of calcium. Three hundred children of this community were examined and nearly 90 per cent had seriously defective teeth; 69 per cent showed affections of the nose and throat, swollen glands, enlarged or diseased tonsils. More than one-third had defective vision, round shoulders, bow legs, or anemia.

Soil

ARE WE STARVING IN A LAND OF PLENTY

Soil experts are warning us today that unless something is done to replenish minerals exhausted from our agricultural lands, we face slow extinction from hidden

Are we Starving to Death?
IN A LAND OF PLENTY
CALCIUM
PHOSPHORUS
MAGNESIUM
SULPHUR
IRON
SICKNESS
SOIL MINERALS DEPLETED AND TIED UP

Jensen's Jetty

Correspondence Course Published Periodically by Dr. Bernard Jensen for Your Protection, Benefit and Enjoyment at 2028 W. Seventh St., Los Angeles, California.

VOL. 1   NO. 3

In this exchange process you will be constantly on the down grade if your life is not constructive day by day. You can think cancer into existence. You can shock diabetes into reality. You can nerve strain an ulcer into the stomach wall. You can coffee and doughnut any cell out of existence in a very short time.

Certainly it is to our advantage that we learn "how to live." Colleges should never graduate a student until he knows how to keep his body well. That would mold our new citizen to his community, occupation or family. With the great storehouse of energy we possess, certainly with a little correct knowledge of bodily upkeep we would remain in good health and enjoy our success after we have attained it.

FROM THE DESK OF DR. JENSEN

I am sure that some of you have thought, especially when you were working on the stomach area, that I put entirely too much emphasis on "Skin Brushing," but just to prove the benefits derived from Skin Brushing I want to tell you of a little experience I had just recently.

A lovely lady in Fresno the other day was waiting to see me on a recheck of her condition, having taken my class and followed my instructions implicitly. While she was waiting for her appointment she watched the girl demonstrate to another patient the proper manner for skin brushing.

One of her first questions to me was to ask why the girl had told the patient to Skin Brush her lower arm, as that part of the arm was displayed to the sun and air and she understood that she was to Skin Brush only the parts of the body that were covered with clothing. I looked at her arm, and she was right in saying that she had been following my instructions implicitly. I could tell at a glance, as she had the upper arm of a twenty year old girl and the forearm of a woman of eighty. It was so obvious, that she went around showing everyone present the difference in the upper part of her arm where she had brushed so diligently and the lower part of the arm. The difference was really remarkable.

Don't forget the Skin Brushing—it really is important.

Dr. Bernard Jensen

SOMETHING TO THINK ABOUT

We are a powerhouse going somewhere to express ourselves. Many of us aren't able to do so much with a sick body. This powerhouse of stored up energy can be used constructively or destructively. The moment it is used to build, harmonize, and construct we are doing the law of God and the law of Nature.

There is no reason for any cell in our body to completely disintegrate without having another one to replace it. It is at this moment when we all want the perfect cell to take the place of the old worn out cell. ...t this moment, however, if the activities of your life ...ave not been along the constructive lines physically, mentally and spiritually you can depend upon it that the new cell will not be a better one.

As Far Back as the Early 1940s, Dr. Jensen's Newsletter Continually Focused on the Essential Relationship Between Soil and Health

Conclusion

In the preceding pages, we have surveyed the varied manifestations of long-term, worldwide pollution, soil depletion, deforestation, and neglect. We have learned how the immune systems of both the Earth and its inhabitants are intimately related to the soil, water, and air. With this understanding, we must begin to meet the challenges we face—for the Earth's sake and for our own.

But, how do we approach this mammoth task? After sixty years of studying health, I feel that I have learned a good deal about reversing toxic conditions in human bodies. I am certain that many of the principles that I employ to reverse the path of human illness will work to cleanse and renew our planet as well. This is because, like our own bodies, the Earth has the ability to cleanse itself. Detoxification is already one of the many normal functions of nature. But, just like an ailing human whose body has been starved of essential nutrients, has been drugged with synthetic chemicals, and has reached the fatigued, multiple-symptom stage, the land, drugged with toxic chemicals, cannot be cleansed properly until we stop adding to its toxic burden.

HUMAN DETOXIFICATION APPLIED TO PLANETARY CLEANSING

According to the dynamic laws of wholistic healing, health is restored when the cause of the problem, rather than its symptoms, is appropriately treated. Therefore, we must approach the decontamination and restoration of the Earth by first identifying the cause of the problem. Then we can start to clean up the water, air, and soil by dealing with that cause and instituting whatever action or program will allow the ensuing healing process to take its course most efficiently and safely.

It is to our advantage that the systems of the planet are interactive—just as each is capable of contaminating the other, they are also capable of healing one another. Again, the principles are similar to those of the human body, and what is beneficial and supportive of one system will benefit the others.

An inspiring example of this is how the living conditions of algae, those miniscule particles of green life inhabiting fresh and salt waters, directly affect the atmosphere. According to information recently published by an independent British team led by scientist James Lovelock, algae in oceans are surrounded by salt that is potentially harmful. The algae protect themselves internally with a harmless salt, *propyl thetin*. That salt, released into the ocean when algae die, is the source of a gas, *dimethyl sulphide*, that promotes the formation of clouds by serving as a "seed" for condensation. No other natural chemical is known to do this. The clouds, in turn, have a beneficial effect on algae; they help stir the wind, which churns up nutrients from lower layers of the ocean. This process demonstrates the natural harmony in which we were meant to live.

We can restore this harmony to our own relationship with nature. But first we must stop pretending that conditions or diseases are "caught" or "just happen." We are not victims.

We do not "catch" diseases. We build them. We have to eat, drink, think, and feel them into existence. We work hard at developing our diseases. We must work just as hard at restoring health.

Similarly, Mother Earth did not "catch" any of her diseases. The ozone layer is not dissolving because of a natural process. Human physical abuse, nothing else, has destroyed this fabric of protective atmosphere. Human chemical abuse in the form of environmental pollution and soil mineral depletion is what must be stopped and reversed in order for the natural healing ability inherent in both the planet and the human being to take over.

RETURN TO SHANGRI-LA

I once took a trip to the Hunza Valley in Pakistan. The Hunza farmers terraced surrounding mountainsides to prevent soil erosion. As Mark discussed, mineral-rich glacial waters feed this soil. As a result, the Hunzas grow beautiful fruits, vegetables, and millet. Throughout my visit there, I could hardly believe the quality of health that I encountered. For example, I met a 140-year-old man whose eyes were clear, whose skin was smooth, and who still had every tooth in his head. I am convinced that diet played a part. The Hunza people ate a little meat, as well as home-grown fruit and vegetables, and drank pure mountain water.

The snows on the Himalaya Mountains kept the Hunza's valley isolated nine months out of the year, so they were not tempted to eat devitalized foods: white flour, white sugar, liquor (except a little homemade wine), and other delicacies of civilization. Interestingly, they also had no need of prisons, police, army, hospitals, dentists, doctors, drugstores, or mental health institutions.

During dinner with the king of Hunza, I noticed that the water he was drinking was cloudy and full of particles. The water served to his guests was clear. I asked him what he was drinking. He told me he drank the water taken straight from the river, containing the glacial silt, because he felt it to be healthier. He didn't think it would be polite, however, to serve such water to his guests. So he served us a clear well water. I was pleased to find in this land that the people's instincts were at least as healthy as their bodies.

The only way for us to return to "Shangri-La," to the natural world, is to stop creating the mess we're in, and to clean up the mess we've made. There is a great deal of research and knowledge about ways to do this, research and knowledge developed by individuals and recorded in books across the world. As Mark reported, the answers are known. Unfortunately, these solutions are rarely implemented on a large scale.

TODD PROVES THAT NATURE HEALS

Let's look at the work of John Todd, founder of the New Alchemy Institute in Cape Cod, Massachusetts, His work illustrates what we are capable of if we only avail ourselves of the information right under our noses. Todd proves that nature is able to detoxify and restore balance, even when contaminated with dangerous, highly toxic chemicals. He designs and runs sewage-treatment plants. But, instead of using deadly chemicals to purify the water of waste, he uses plants, fish, and other aquatic life. Todd says

> Since the [passage of the] Clean Water Act in 1972, we've spent billions of dollars and haven't really improved water quality. We use 70,000 different chemicals routinely in commerce and then dump them into the water. Those chemicals are ungluing the natural world.
>
> The waste-treatment industry is getting scary. To meet regulations on some chemicals, we use others that aren't regulated. We use chlorine to meet ammonia standards, and in the process make chloroform and chloramine, which don't have standards. To get rid of phosphate, we precipitate it out with aluminum. Aluminum is toxic in all parts of the environment, but we haul it out of sewage-treatment plants and dump it onto the land by the ton. We use high concentrations of copper salts, which are not natural in ecosystems, to get rid of algae, which are.
>
> Every time the restrictions on one pollutant get stronger, the chemicals to remove it get stronger. That

can't be the right way to go. It must be possible to use sunshine and ecology to purify water—as nature does.

John Todd knows that nature handles every kind of waste by turning it into a nutrient. For example, soil and water are full of bacteria that transforms ammonia into nitrate, a plant food. Nitrate is absorbed by plants, which are eaten by animals, which excrete ammonia again to keep the cycle going. It's part of the nitrogen cycle, one of the great biogeochemical cycles of the planet. This is the cycle upon which Todd bases the designs of his treatment plants.

Todd received training about plants with purifying abilities from Kathe Seidel at the Max Planck Institute in West Germany. Although reliance on cleanup techniques is not the answer we seek, cleanup techniques such as these are excellent, proven methods we can use until we can completely stop the cause of the pollution.

Once we end the chemical flood that is poisoning our planet by halting all sources of pollution and toxic increase; by cleaning up the air, soil, and water as well as we can; and by isolating excessively toxic areas; we need to identify inherent weaknesses on the face of our planet and give them special care so they return to health and productivity.

THE EARTH NEEDS TO BE FED

In a human being, inherently weak organs, glands, or tissues are slower and less efficient in assimilating nutrients and in eliminating wastes than stronger, healthier tissue. Therefore, unless they are fed with the nutrient elements they need, they easily become fatigued and unable to detoxify as well. Soon they are overloaded with waste from the bloodstream as well as their own metabolic byproducts.

What are the comparable "inherently weak" areas of the Earth? They are underground repositories of water (aquifers) that should be kept pure. They are rivers, lakes, and seas that are exposed to human activity but also serve as food and drinking water sources. They are soils, such as tropical and subtropical varieties, that are more delicate. They are forests that protect important watersheds and serve as barriers to erosion. They are prairies and other broad flat lands that are vulnerable to wind erosion. We might include highly toxified areas such as Chernobyl, in the U.S.S.R., and the republic of Vietnam, where Agent Orange and other chemical defoliants were used liberally.

Just as acidic toxins in the body can be chemically neutralized using sodium, potassium, calcium, magnesium, and manganese, we should be able to find chemicals that neutralize some of the highly toxic areas of the world. Of course, I realize that nothing now known can "neutralize" radioactivity. The best we can do with radioactive contamination is to contain it, to protect people from going near it, and to stop creating it.

ORGANIC FARMING WORKS

Many more methods of cleaning up the environment will be researched and developed as we decide to learn from nature. My organic farming experiences have served to teach me the importance of learning through listening and observing. I have found the art of farming simply to be the art of any partnership—listening, observing, and responding. Listen to inner wisdom, listen to your partner, observe everything. The partnership with nature, if we listen and observe, teaches us the mysteries of creation. How often have we wondered how is it that nature can create a baby? Well, how is it that nature can create a carrot? The way is taught to us when we join in partnership with nature.

By observing and listening—often to other farmers with experience—I learned how to interpret insect problems as imbalance of soil chemistry. I learned how to respond to this problem using natural controls such as soaps, soils, botanical insecticides (such as garlic juice), microbial insecticides, cover mulches, companion planting with insect repellent plants such as marigolds, trap crops, ladybugs for aphid control, and praying mantises to control other insects.

In place of chemical fertilizers, I use compost, green manures, animal manures, worm castings, fish meal, blood meal, bone meal, and seaweed. Rock fertilizers or lime may be added to the soil to alter acidity or to provide a slow, steady release of nutrients.

WORMS: NATURE'S SOIL BUILDERS

Do not be surprised at which of its creatures nature empowers to help humankind. The lowly earthworm, for example, is one of our greatest hopes for the restoration of our country's vanishing topsoil. Earthworms belong to the soil community. The soil is their home, their source of food, their protection. In return for the soil's hospitality, worms break down organic matter in the soil, and may deposit as much as seven to eighteen tons per year of nitrogen-rich excretory castings on a single acre. These castings, which also contain concentrations of many of the chemical elements needed by the soil, form a major contribution to renewal of topsoil. We should know all we can about worms before we ever start gardening or farming.

When we make our own fertilizer by composting, worms help to break down the compost faster. Worm castings contain five times the amount of nitrogen, seven times the phosphate content, and eleven times more potash than the material the worm consumed. This is, of course, a very rich and desirable fertilizer.

These hard-working helpers build soil in other ways, as well. The burrowing action of worms aerates the soil, keeps it drained, and aids the penetration of plant roots. The English evolutionist Charles Darwin studied worms and documented how they transport soil by bringing it to the surface from below in quantities that amount to several tons per acre, annually. At the same time, they consume, draw into their burrows, and incorporate into the soil as much as twenty pounds per square yard of organic matter every six months. Darwin estimated that worms could create an inch to an inch and a half of topsoil in ten years.

If an earthworm can avoid being eaten or overexposed to light, it may live as long as six years. I believe we need to have a "worm renaissance" on our over-chemicalized agricultural land to restore the life that is characteristic of healthy soil.

Worms Need Good Food

However, worms cannot do it alone. Worms cannot make mineral-rich castings out of mineral-deficient food. If earthworms are fed grass clippings completely lacking in calcium, their castings will be equally lacking in calcium. When the organic matter we use in our compost piles is chemically deficient, we may have to go outside our local areas to get the properly mineralized organic material to add to the soil in order to restore the chemicals it is lacking. Of course, we should get a chemical analysis of our soil to make sure we are adding only those things that are truly needed and desirable.

To make sure we have the proper balance in our compost, we should add some rotted animal manure, bought or traded from a chicken or turkey farm, or from a riding stable, or from some other source, such as a rabbit farm. Goat manure is excellent because it does not draw flies. Seaweed is an excellent source of iodine and trace minerals. Seaweed is added by trench composting, or by spreading on the surface and discing into the soil. Seaweed is an important addition to any compost pile. Lime, gypsum, dolomite, and phosphate rock can be added if necessary. There are specially prepared, multi-mineral rock fertilizers manufactured for the organic farmer.

While these measures will help on a small-scale basis, we must not fool ourselves that this is enough. Unless we clean up our planet and revise our attitude toward agriculture and soil, all this knowledge will be wasted. If the trend continues unbridled, it is quite likely that we will starve to death at some point in the near future.

Two-thirds of the people in the world go to bed hungry every night. There is famine in Africa. In Asia, where more than half the world's population is concentrated, food shortages are a way of life. Hundreds of disease-resistant varieties of native rice have been lost as traditional farming techniques have been replaced with high-tech farming methods imported from the West. Meanwhile, tractors lie rusting in the fields because Asian farmers cannot afford the fuel to run them or the agricultural chemicals needed to grow hybrid plants. The result is starvation.

Rich western nations do not lack calories. They do lack true nourishment. Therefore, they have a serious problem with malnutrition and the diseases caused or influenced by malnutrition. In the final analysis, malnutrition is just another form of starvation.

In all forms of starvation, the immune system is injured and disease increases. I do not believe that AIDS could exist today if there was not such a great weakening of the immune system brought about by the use of drugs, exposure to pollution, and poor food habits.

END SELF-POLLUTION

I once had a woman patient with a running sore on her forehead that had developed several months before. The treatment she had received did not help. I noticed that she dyed her hair. When I examined her eyes, I saw reflex indications of drug deposits in her head and scalp areas. I told her that she had to stop using the hair dye.

She became very upset and refused. She was married, it seemed, to a man sixteen years younger than she was; and she was afraid of his reaction if he saw her gray hair. I asked, "Don't you have something more to hold your marriage together than the color of your hair?" She did not like the idea of not dying her hair, and she left.

Several months later, she came back with the same problem and agreed to do anything I asked. I asked her to stop dying her hair, and I put her on an elimination diet. Within two months, the sore was completely healed.

Like the woman in the preceding example, many of us do not realize the extent to which we are polluting ourselves with chemicals—hair dyes, hair sprays, permanent wave solutions, deodorants, antiperspirants, makeup, aftershave lotions, colognes, perfumes, bubble baths, room deodorizers, soaps, household cleaning solutions, chlorine bleach. We can name dozens more—and this would only begin to touch on the thousands of chemicals we use each day.

Confirmation that these cause changes in health abounds. People who work around the chemicals used in photo labs often have to change jobs for health reasons. Painters who work with lead-based paints and artists who work with leaded stained-glass windows often develop lead poisoning.

We breathe chemical pollution in the air. We drink it in the water. We apply it to our skin. We eat it in our foods. We subject our children, our pets, and our loved ones to poisons about which we have little knowledge. We have chemicals everywhere. We do not realize what they are doing to us and to all living creatures.

Unless we develop guidelines for chemicals and their use that safeguard our environment and our health, we are moving in a dangerous direction. We must stop the chemical flood unleashed in the name of progress and prosperity. We need to reconsider our overemphasis on drugs and symptom-suppressant approaches to health care. We need to look to nature for alternatives to both. We must choose life over greed.

LEARN FROM MISTAKES OF THE PAST

There have been many reasons for the decline and fall of great civilizations. The demise of the Mayan civilization 600 years before Spanish explorers arrived in the Americas has long been considered a mystery. The majestic monuments, pyramids, and temples they built testify to a culture that thrived for 1,500 years. What factors contributed to its destruction? According to one expert, the Mayans' need for food and fuel exhausted the land they lived on. It is clear to us, after reading the previous pages of this book, that there is one catalyst that ultimately exhausts land and renders it incapable of sustaining life. That catalyst is human ignorance—the refusal to take notice—of how to care for the soil.

If the great nations of the world truly desire peace above all else, then let them turn to this great work. For the work of restoration of planetary health does not pit us against each other; rather, it binds us together: planet, human, animal, plant, and microbe. If the great nations of the world truly desire health and prosperity for their citizens, this is the work that will employ all; this is the work that will heal all. But you and I cannot wait for governments to decide. We must each do our part to return nourishment to Mother Earth even as we take nourishment from her.

As we work together to help nature to become cleaner, and our air, water, and soil quality is restored, we will witness the birth of a new world civilization in which the integrity of nature; the integrity of life; the integrity of body, mind, and morality in humankind is full of interdependent health, prosperity, and peace. I urge you to work toward the day when we can celebrate attainment of this worthy goal.

Appendix
Selected Bibliography

Books

Abbey, Edward. *Down the River With Henry Thoreau, 1st Ed.* Salt Lake City: G. M. Smith, 1981.

Abrahamson, E. M., and Pezet, A. W. *Body, Mind and Sugar.* New York: Holt, Rhinehart and Winston, 1951.

Andersen, Arden B. *Life and Energy in Agriculture.* Kansas City, MO: Acres, USA Publishing, 1989.

Asher, Carl. *Bacteria, Inc.* Boston: Bruce Humphries, 1949.

Balfour, E. B. *The Living Soil.* New York: The Devin-Adair Company, 1943.

Ballantine, Rudolph. *Diet and Nutrition: A Holistic Approach.* Honesdale, PA: Himalayan International Institute, 1978.

Ballantine, Rudolph. *Transition to Vegetarianism.* Honesdale, PA: Himalayan International Institute, 1987.

Beddoe, A. F. *Biological Ionization as Applied to Farming and Soil Management.* Bragg, CA: Agri-Bio Systems, 1986.

Bicknell, Franklin, and Prescott, Frederick. *The Vitamins in Medicine, 3rd Ed.* Palmyra, WI: Lee Foundation for Nutritional Research, 1953.

Blate, Michael. *The Tao of Health.* Davie, FL: Falkynor Books, 1978.

Carson, Rachel L. *Silent Spring.* Greenwich, CT: Crest Books, 1962.

Dadd, Debra Lynn. *Nontoxic and Natural*. Los Angeles: Jeremy Tarcher, 1984.

Dufty, William. *Sugar Blues*. Radner, PA: Chilton Book Company, 1975.

Encyclopaedia Brittanica. 1899 ed., s.v. "von Leibig, Justus." Chicago: Encyclopaedia Brittanica, Inc.

Erasmus, Udo. *Fats and Oils: The Complete Guide to Fats and Oils in Health and Nutrition*. Vancouver, BC: Aliva Books, 1986.

Fukuoka, Masanobu. *The One-Straw Revolution*. Emmaus, PA: Rodale Press, 1978.

Graham, Sylvester. *Treatise on Bread and Bread Making*. Boston: Light and Stearns, 1837.

Griffin, La Dean. *Health in the Space Age*. Orem, UT: Biworld Publishers, 1982.

Gross, Martin L. *The Doctors*. New York: Random House, 1966.

Grossinger, Richard. *Planet Medicine*. Berkeley, CA: North Atlantic Books, 1985.

Grun, Bernard. *The Timetables of History*. New York: Simon & Schuster, 1982.

Guyton, A. *Textbook of Medical Physiology, 6th ed*. Philadelphia: W. B. Saunders, 1981.

Harrower, Henry R. *Practical Endocrinology, 2nd ed*. Palmyra, WI: Lee Foundation for Nutritional Research, 1932.

Hamaker, John D., and Weaver, Donald. *The Survival of Civilization*. Burlingame, CA: Hamaker-Weaver Publishers, 1982.

Hauschka, Rudolph. *Nutrition*. London: Steiner Press, 1983.

Hensel, Julius. *Bread From Stones*. Germany, 1892.

Howard, Albert. *An Agricultural Testament*. London: Oxford University Press, 1940.

Howell, Edward. *Enzyme Nutrition*. Garden City, NY: Avery Publishing Group, 1985.

Idso, Sherwood. *CO₂ and Global Change: Earth in Transition.* Tempe, AZ: IBR Press, 1989.

Inlander, Charles, Levin, Lowell, and Weiner, Ed. *Medicine on Trial.* Englewood Cliffs, NJ: Prentice Hall Press, 1988.

Jarvis, D. C. *Folk Medicine.* New York: Holt, Rinehart & Winston, 1958.

Jensen, Bernard. *Foods That Heal.* Garden City Park, NY: Avery Publishing Group, 1988.

Johnson, Leland G. *Biology.* Dubuque, IA: Wm. C. Brown Company, 1983.

Kirk, David. *Biology, The Unity and Diversity of Life.* Belmont, CA: Wadsworth Publishing Company, 1978.

Kirshmann, John D., and Dunne, Lavon J. *Nutrition Almanac, 2nd ed.* New York: McGraw-Hill Book Company, 1984.

Koop, Everett C., and the United States Department of Health and Human Services, Public Health Service. *The Surgeon General's Report on Nutrition and Health.* Rocklin, CA: Prima Publishing, 1988.

Lambert, Gille. *Conquest of Age: The Extraordinary Story of Dr. Paul Niehaus.* New York: Rinehart & Company, 1959.

Logsgon, Gene. *Better Soil.* Emmaus, PA: Rodale Press, 1975.

Martin, Vance, and Inglis, Mary, eds. *Wilderness: The Way Ahead.* Forres, Scotland: Findhorn Press, 1984.

Mason, Marion, et al. *Nutrition and the Cell: The Inside Story.* Chicago: Year Book Medical Publishers, Inc., 1973.

Maxwell, Kenneth E. *Environment of Life, 3rd Ed.* Monterey, CA: Brooks/Cole Publishing Company, 1980.

McArdle, William D., Katch, Frank I., and Katch, Victor L. *Exercise Physiology: Energy, Nutrition, and Human Performance. 2nd ed.* Philadelphia: Lea & Febiger, 1986.

McCarrison, Robert. *Studies in Deficiency Diseases.* London: Oxford Medical Publications, 1921.

Myers, Norman. *GAIA: An Atlas of Planetary Management*. Garden City, NY: Anchor Press/Doubleday, 1984.

Natenberg, Maurice. *The Legacy of Doctor Wiley*. Chicago: Regent House, 1957.

Netter, Frank H. *The Ciba Collection Number 4: The Endocrine System*. Edison, NJ: Ciba Company, 1965.

Odum, Eugene P. *Fundamentals of Ecology, 2nd Ed*. Philadelphia and London: W. B. Saunders Company, 1959.

Pearce, Ian. *The Wholistic Approach to Cancer*. Dunbartonshire, England: Famedram Publishing, Ltd., 1983.

Peshek, Robert J. *Nutrition for a Healthy Heart*. Riverside, CA: Color Codes Systems, 1979.

Price, Weston A. *Nutrition and Physical Degeneration*. San Diego: Price-Pottenger Nutrition Foundation, 1939.

Quigley, D. T. *The National Malnutrition, 3rd Ed*. Palmyra, WI: Lee Foundation for Nutritional Research, 1943.

Randolph, Therons G. *Human Ecology and Susceptibility to the Chemical Environment*. Seventh printing. Springfield, IL: Charles Thomas Books, 1962.

Rodale, J. I., and Staff. *The Complete Book of Food and Nutrition*. Emmaus, PA: Rodale Books, 1961.

Rubel, Lovis L. *The GP and the Endocrine Glands*. Decatur, IL: 1959.

Tannahill, Reay. *Food in History*. Briarcliff Manor, NY: Stein and Day, 1973.

Thomas, Lewis. *The Medusa and the Snail*. New York: Viking Press, 1979.

Thompson, William. *Medicines From the Earth*. New York: Alfred van der Marck Editions, 1978.

United States Department of Health and Human Services. *The Surgeon General's Report on Nutrition and Health*. New York: St. Martin's Press, July, 1988.

van der Post, Laurens. *Walk With A White Bushman*. New York: William Morrow and Company, Inc., 1986.

von Liebig, Justus. *Agricultural Chemistry*. Germany: 1855.

von Liebig, Justus. *The Natural Laws of Husbandry*. Germany: c. 1870.

Waksman, Selman. *My Life With Microbes*. New York: Simon & Schuster, 1954.

Watt, Kenneth. *Annual Review of the Environment*. Chicago: Encyclopaedia Brittanica, Inc., 1988.

Werback, Melvyn R. *Nutritional Influences on Illness*. New Canaan, CT: Keats Publishing, 1988.

Wheelwright, Edith Grey. *Medicinal Plants and Their History*. New York: Dover Publications, 1935.

Wigmore, Ann, and Earp-Thomas, G. H. *Organic Soil: A New Concept in Diet*. Boston: Rising Sun Publications, 1978.

Wiley, Harvey W. *The History of a Crime Against the Food Law*. Washington, DC: 1929.

Williams, Roger J. *Physicians' Handbook on Orthomolecular Medicine*. New York: Pergamon Press, 1977.

Williams, Sue Rodale. *Nutrition and Diet Therapy, 5th Ed*. St. Louis: Times/Mirror Mosby College, 1979.

Wolf, Max, and Ransberger, Carl. *Enzyme Therapy*. Los Angeles: Regent House, 1972.

Wrench, W. T. *The Wheel of Health*. London: C. W. Daniel Company, Ltd., 1938.

Yepsen, Roger, Jr., and the editors of *Organic Gardening and Farming* magazine. *Organic Plant Protection*. Emmaus, PA: Rodale Press, 1976.

Congressional Reports and Hearings

U.S. Congress. House of Representatives. Select Committee. *Investigation of the Use of Chemicals in Food Products*, 81st Congress, 2nd session, 1950.

U.S. Congress. Senate. Select Committee, Senator George McGovern, Chairman. *Diet Related to Killer Diseases V Nutrition and Mental Health*, 95th Congress, 1st session, 22 June 1977.

Government Documents

United States Department of Agriculture. *Food and Life*. 1939, pp. 238–239.

United States Food and Drug Administration. Department of Health and Human Services. *Food Defect Action Levels*. 1988.

Journal Articles

(A discussion of the relationship between Alzheimer's disease and aluminum.) *The Lancet* (14 January 1989).

Balling, R. C. "Historical Temperature Trends in the United States and the Effects of Urban Population Growth." *Journal of Geophysical Research* (20 March 1989).

Birchall, J. D., and Chappell, J. S. "Aluminum, Chemical Physiology, and Alzheimer's Disease." *The Lancet* (29 October 1988).

Heylin, Michael, ed. "Fluoridation." *Chemical & Engineering News* (1 August 1988).

Hileman, Bette. "Special Report: Fluoridation of Water: Questions About Health Risks and Benefits Remain After More Than Forty Years." *Chemical & Engineering News* (1 August 1988).

Morgan, Agnes Fay. "The Effect of Imbalance in the 'Filtrate Fraction' of the Vitamin B Complex in Dogs." *Science* (14 March 1941).

Roger, Regnault C. "The Nutritional Incidence of Flavonoids: Some Physiological and Metabolic Considerations." *Experientia* (15 September 1988): pp. 725–804.

Schimmel, Elihu M. "The Hazards of Hospitalization." *Annals of Internal Medicine* (January 1964): pp. 100–110.

Seifter, Eli. (A discussion of the relationship between Vitamin A and the thymus.) *Journal of Infectious Diseases* (September 1975).

Laws

United States Food and Drug Administration. *Federal Food, Drug and Cosmetic Act as Amended and Related Law.* Rockville, MD: United States Department of Health and Human Services, 1985.

Magazine Articles

Harris, Louis & Assoc. (Harris Poll shows public prefers organic food.) *Organic Gardening,* November 1988.

Kahn, Carol. "Freeze Your Immunity." *Longevity,* November 1988.

"Living Room Lung Cancer." *American Health Magazine,* June 1988.

Mann, John David. "Bread From Stones." *Solstice,* May 1988.

Mann, John David. "Perspective on Health and The Environment." *Solstice.*

Meadows, Donella H. "The New Alchemist." *Harrowsmith.* November/December 1988.

"Nine States Confirm Aflatoxin Contamination." *Time.* 31 October 1988.

Oak Ridge Associated Universities. "Eco-Update." *Acres, USA,* April 1989.

"Taking the Earth's Vital Signs: NASA Seeks to Become a Major Force in the Campaign to Save the Planet." *Time,* 5 June 1989.

Tennakone, K., and Wickramanayake, S. "Aluminum Leaching From Cooking Utensils." *Nature.*

Newspaper Articles

Accola, John. "Mother Earth a Real Danger to Pregnancies." *Rocky Mountain News,* 29 March 1989, p. 51.

Anderson, Mark. "Christians Are Wasting Millions of Trees." *Denver Post*, 2 December 1988, p. 7(B).

Brooke, James. "Brazil Wants Aid to Fight Pollution, But No Strings," *New York Times*, 21 March 1989.

"Fluoridation Politics Makes Bad Science." *Christian Science Monitor*, 23 August 1988.

Ingersoll, Bruce. "Tough Environment." *Wall Street Journal*, 20 January 1989.

"Logging Threatens Oldest U.S. Forest Land." *New York Times*. Reprinted with permission in the *Denver Post*, 20 March 1989.

Meier, Barry. "Poison Produce." *Wall Street Journal*, 26 March 1987.

Nelson, Elmer M. (Comments in federal testimony by Elmer M. Nelson, M.D., head, United States Food and Drug Administration, Division of Nutrition.) *Washington Post*, 26 October 1949.

"Spreading Poison; Fungus in Corn Crop, A Potent Carcinogen, Invades Food Supplies; Regulators Fail to Stop Sales of Last Fall's Harvest Laden With Aflatoxin." *Wall Street Journal*, 23 February 1989.

"Statistics on Birth Defects." *Newsweek*, and *Birth Defects Branch, Centers for Disease Control, Atlanta*. Reprinted with permission in the *Rocky Mountain News*, 29 March 1989.

Pamphlets

Mineralization. Savage, Albert Carter. Nicholasville, KY, 1942.

Portfolios

Lee, Royal. *Assorted manuscripts and articles: 1923–1963*. Palmyra, WI: Lee Foundation for Nutritional Research.

Lee, Royal. Reprinted material from *The Agriculturalist, The Doctor, The Homemaker*. Palmyra, WI: Lee Foundation for Nutritional Research.

Reports

Davidson, J. R. *Cancer: A Nutritional Deficiency.* Manitoba, Canada: University of Manitoba Science Department, (1943).

United States Department of Health and Human Services. *Surgeon General's Report on Nutrition and Health.* Rocklin, CA: Prima Publishing & Communication, (1988).

Statistics

United States Bureau of Census, *Statistical Abstract of the United States,* Washington, DC, 1937.

United States Bureau of Census, *Statistical Abstract of the United States,* Washington, DC, 1960.

United States Bureau of Census, *Statistical Abstract of the United States,* Washington, DC, 1987.

Studies

Yale-New Haven Hospital Study. See: Journal Articles section. Schimmel, Elihu M. "The Hazards of Hospitalization." *Annals of Internal Medicine.*

Transcribed Lectures

Albrecht, William. *Assorted lectures.* Fort Collins, CO: Selene River Press.

Lee, Royal. *Assorted Lectures: 1923–1963.* Palmyra, WI: Lee Foundation for Nutritional Research.

Lee, Royal. *Lectures on Malnutrition: 1923–1963.* Fort Collins, CO: Selene River Press.

Videotapes

Dr. Pottenger's Cat Experiments. San Diego: Price-Pottenger Nutrition Foundation.

Dr. Price's Search for Health. San Diego: Price-Pottenger Nutrition Foundation.

Stopping the Coming Ice Age. Berkeley, CA: People for a Future. 1988.

Index

About the Authors

Dr. Bernard Jensen

One of America's foremost pioneering nutritionists, Dr. Bernard Jensen began his career in 1929 as a chiropractic physician. He soon turned to the art of nutrition in search of remedies for his own health problems. In his formative years, Dr. Jensen studied under such giants as Dr. Benedict Lust, Dr. John Tilden, Dr. John H. Kellogg, and Dr. V.G. Rocine. Later, he observed firsthand the cultural practices of people in more than fifty-five countries, discovering important links between food and health. In 1955, Dr. Jensen established the Hidden Valley Ranch in Escondido, California as a retreat and learning center dedicated to the healing principles of nature.

Over the years, Dr. Jensen has received a multitude of prestigious awards and honors for his work in the healing arts. These honors include Knighthood in the Order of St. John of Malta, the Dag Hammarskjold Peace Award of Belgium, and an award from

Queen Juliana of the Netherlands. He is also the author of numerous articles and bestselling books. At age eighty-three, he continues to teach, travel, and learn.

Mark Anderson

A recognized authority on the topics of global ecology and wholistic health, Mark Anderson has spent much of the past eighteen years traveling the world to study and teach clinical nutrition from the soil up. His stimulating and informative lectures on traditional diets, health patterns of native peoples, and agriculture have been featured at seminars and conferences in Africa, Asia, Europe, and India, as well as throughout the United States and Canada. Mark's articles about natural approaches to nutrition and health have been published in scores of professional health journals in the United States.

A sought-after guest on radio and television, Mark continues to lecture at seminars and conferences nationwide. New York born and raised, and educated at the University of Denver, Mark now makes his home on a Colorado ranch, which he shares with his wife, Stephanie, and son, Ethan.